DOING THE RIGHT THING

DOING THE RIGHT THING

*Taking Care of
Your Elderly Parents
Even If They Didn't
Take Care of You*

Roberta Satow, Ph.D.

JEREMY P. TARCHER / PENGUIN
A MEMBER OF PENGUIN GROUP (USA) INC.
NEW YORK

JEREMY P. TARCHER/PENGUIN

Published by the Penguin Group

Penguin Group (USA) Inc., 375 Hudson Street, New York, New York 10014, USA • Penguin Group
(Canada), 10 Alcorn Avenue, Toronto, Ontario M4V 3B2, Canada (a division of Pearson Penguin
Canada Inc.) • Penguin Books Ltd, 80 Strand, London WC2R 0RL, England • Penguin Ireland,
25 St Stephen's Green, Dublin 2, Ireland (a division of Penguin Books Ltd) • Penguin Group (Australia),
250 Camberwell Road, Camberwell, Victoria 3124, Australia (a division of Pearson Australia Group Pty
Ltd) • Penguin Books India Pvt Ltd, 11 Community Centre, Panchsheel Park, New Delhi–110 017,
India • Penguin Group (NZ), Cnr Airborne and Rosedale Roads, Albany, Auckland 1310,
New Zealand (a division of Pearson New Zealand Ltd) • Penguin Books (South Africa) (Pty) Ltd,
24 Sturdee Avenue, Rosebank, Johannesburg 2196, South Africa

Penguin Books Ltd, Registered Offices: 80 Strand, London WC2R 0RL, England

This book is designed to provide accurate and authoritative information in regard to the subject matter
covered, and every effort has been made to ensure that it is correct and complete. However, neither the
publisher nor the author is engaged in rendering professional advice or services to the individual
reader, and this book is not intended as a substitute for advice from a trained counselor, therapist, or
other similar professional. If you require such advice or other expert assistance, you should seek the
services of a competent professional in the appropriate specialty.

While the author has made every effort to provide accurate telephone numbers and Internet addresses at
the time of publication, neither the publisher nor the author assumes any responsibility for errors, or for
changes that occur after publication.

Most Tarcher/Penguin books are available at special quantity discounts for bulk purchase for sales
promotions, premiums, fund-raising, and educational needs. Special books or book excerpts also can be
created to fit specific needs. For details, write Penguin Group (USA) Inc. Special Markets, 375 Hudson
Street, New York, NY 10014.

Library of Congress Cataloging-in-Publication Data

Satow, Roberta.
    Doing the right thing : taking care of your elderly parents
even if they didn't take care of you / Roberta Satow.
        p.   cm.
    Includes bibliographical references and index.
    ISBN 1-58542-392-0
    1. Aging parents—United States.   2. Aging parents—Care—United States.   3. Adult children
of aging parents—United States.   4. Intergenerational relations—United States.   5. Caregivers—
United States.   I. Title.
HQ1063.6.S28   2005   2004058870
306.874'084'6—dc22

Printed in the United States of America
10   9   8   7   6   5   4   3   2   1

This book is printed on acid-free paper. ♾

Book design by Lovedog Studio

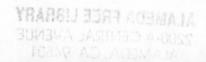

For Richard, Matthew and Jason

CONTENTS

Acknowledgments   ix

Preface   xi

Introduction   I

Part *I*. The Internal Struggle

Chapter One
Setting Limits   27

Chapter Two
Getting Angry and Getting Over It   55

Chapter Three
Feeling Guilty and Forgiving Yourself   84

**Part II. Relationships That Offer Support
or Create Conflict**

Chapter Four
Spouses   115

Chapter Five
Siblings   140

Part III. Ethnicity and Gender

Chapter Six
Cultural Scripts for Caregivers   165

Chapter Seven
Daughters   189

Chapter Eight
Sons   218

Conclusion
How Can I Handle This Better?   244

Notes   253

Bibliography   260

Index   265

ACKNOWLEDGMENTS

My agent, Gail Hochman, believed in this book from the moment she read the first draft of my proposal. I will always be grateful to her. Mitch Horowitz has been a wonderful editor, offering his support and good judgment throughout.

Geri DeLuca, Jennifer McCormick and, more recently, Nancy Hoch read chapters and revisions of chapters endlessly. They believed in me and they made me believe in my writing. They always heard my voice and encouraged me to strengthen it and let it ring out.

My sister, Florence Isaacs, and friends Jo Dobkin and Randy Lehrer read several chapters and offered helpful comments. My husband, Richard Wool, and sons, Matthew and Jason, suffered through my obsessing about the book for over three years.

I could not have done my interviews with caregivers without the help of Anne Potter, director of Senior Citizen Services, and Nancy Lindoerfer, Senior Services counselor for the town of New Milford, Connecticut; and Bonnie Walson, executive director of Heritage Day Health Centers in Columbus, Ohio. They offered their offices for interviewing caregivers and did everything they could to make my research possible.

Most of all I would like to thank the caregivers who opened their hearts to me and shared their loving feelings as well as their pain. Thank you all.

PREFACE

THIS BOOK IS PERSONAL. It is about middle-aged caregiving as a stressful stage of life that many of us—myself included—are confronting, but for which we are often unprepared. In it, I talk about my feelings about my mother and father as well as other people's feelings about their parents. I discuss the struggle to be conscious and not fall back into old patterns—what psychoanalysts call "the repetition compulsion." You may ask yourself: How can she help me when she has these feelings herself? How can she help me when she is just like me—struggling against the compulsion to repeat old patterns?

I have asked myself these questions—and others. Should I write like an authority who is above having these conflicts and struggles so that the reader can feel confidence in me? Or should I disclose personal material that my patients and readers may see and that may affect their feelings about me? I have struggled with all these questions—yours and mine—

while I was writing this book. I came to the conclusion that disclosing my own struggles was worth the risk because I am trying to communicate that the struggle described here is an ongoing one.

There is no one day after which we no longer have to contend with the compulsion to repeat old patterns that keep us stuck and unhappy. A major theme of the book is that old patterns and conflicts that remain either unresolved or incompletely resolved reemerge throughout our lives—especially during stressful times such as caregiving. If we do not resolve them, the best we can do is reach a point where we are more conscious of the telltale signs that presage their reemergence. We can get to a point at which a red flag goes up when we are about to plunge into the depths of despair like a helpless child; when we are about to do something self-destructive; or when we are about to say something hurtful. We can get to a point at which we can realize the meaning of what we just said or did and not let our lives or our selves get out of control. Or we can do even better than that. We can resolve the underlying conflicts that cause us to repeat painful experiences.

I could not write this book as if I did not also have these struggles, share these feelings and struggle to resolve underlying conflicts. Therapists and patients are not qualitatively different types of people, but simply people at different stages in the quest for consciousness and resolution. I tell my patients that putting their feelings into words makes their feelings more conscious and makes them less likely to act them out in ways they will regret. In this book I have tried to put my feelings, and those of the caregivers I interviewed, into words for those people who have not been entirely able to do so themselves.

Some of the fifty caregivers I interviewed for this book had done or were doing a substantial amount of work to become more conscious about what they were experiencing in the process of caregiving. They were able to resolve some old issues with their parents and experienced caregiving as an important stage in their own emotional development. Others were unable to move beyond entrenched patterns. I want to thank all of them for sharing their conflicts, love, wishes, fears, anger, guilt and hope with me. I found their stories compelling, and knowing each and every one of them has enriched my life and the experience I have been able to bring to this book. Their names and identifying traits have been altered to protect their privacy.

INTRODUCTION

IT'S 7 P.M. AND I HAVE just walked into the house after a weekend away in the country. As I put all my packages down, I notice that my son Jason has left a message for me: "Grandma's in the hospital again." I feel alternately mad at her for ruining my evening (I'm so hungry), bad for her that she's alone and probably feeling out of control, frightened that she is dying, and furious that she's probably *not* dying— just nauseated again. I think to myself that soon 911 will be saying: "Oh, it's Sarah again." I have to go or I won't be able to stand myself, but I hate to drive alone at night and my husband, Richard, has just driven three hours from Connecticut in traffic and I don't want to ask him to drive me. I call my sister in hopes that she will come with me instead. When I call she says her husband thinks he has a blood clot in his leg again. He has to go to the hospital and probably will have to cancel his business trip. I can hear the anxiety in her voice. To my great relief, Richard offers to drive me to see my mother.

An hour later I find my mother in the emergency room at Maimonides Hospital in Brooklyn. It's familiar to me. The room is full of Hasidic Jews and Hispanics with nurses and aides milling around. I look through all the curtains set up around the nurses' station until I find her. She is opposite the cubicle where I found my father at 11 p.m. on the rainy night before he died. "Hi, Mom," I greet her, and she smiles at me. Part of me is angry at her because I came all this way and didn't eat dinner and she's smiling at me. "I thought I had a heart attack," she says, "but I didn't. I had pains in my right arm and with a heart attack it's your left arm." While I am relieved that she didn't have a heart attack, I am also furious that I came all this way and she *didn't* even have a heart attack! What kind of daughter am I?

Uncle Morris, my mother's brother-in-law, is standing next to my mother's bed in the cubicle. He lives in the same apartment building as my mother and called 911; he came with her in the ambulance. "Hi, Uncle Morris. Thanks for bringing Mom here," I greet him. "Have you had dinner?" No, he tells me, but waves as if to say: I'm all right, don't worry. But if I'm not going to have dinner, I'll be even angrier if he stays here too and there would have been no reason for me to come. So I thank him and Richard walks him to the bus down the block. After Morris and Richard leave, my mother says casually: "You know, I think Morris has my keys," and starts shuffling through her purse. Sure enough she doesn't have her keys. I realize that my mother, who is not likely to be discharged until after Morris is asleep, won't be able to get into her apartment. I start running to the bus stop to try to reach Morris, but he is gone by the time I get there and I am left gasping for breath.

I find Richard back in the waiting room and tell him the sad story. "Don't worry," he reassures me, "you can call him in a little while and ask him to leave the keys for you." But there's no place for Morris to leave them because there's no doorman in their building. We will have to get the keys from Morris and return to the hospital. After half an hour I call Morris on my cell phone, but he isn't home. I keep redialing until I notice the sign: "No cell phones." Maybe it causes someone's pacemaker to skip or something. I start wondering if I've unwittingly killed someone here with my phone. I go looking for a pay phone and call. Finally, Morris is home and I tell him I've been calling a long time. He says he stopped to get a bite to eat, but I can come now and get the keys.

Richard and I drive to Morris and my mother's building. Richard waits in the car. I sprint up the three flights of stairs because I'm too nervous to wait for the elevator. I ring the bell and . . . no answer. I keep ringing the bell, but there's no answer. How could he not be home? I just called him five minutes ago. Oh, my God, I think to myself, he must have died after I called. He's in there lying on the floor. He's not used to eating so late. Maybe he got so hungry that he had a heart attack. He died of hunger.

He probably didn't die of hunger. Maybe he went out again. So I run down the stairs and find someone at the door. "Did you see Mr. Weiss?" "Yes," he says, "he came in a little while ago." So he's in there, he didn't go out. I sprint up the stairs again and ring the bell and knock on the door concurrently. Still there's no answer. He's a little deaf. Maybe he didn't hear the bell. But probably he's dead. I continue knocking and ringing frantically and start worrying that the neighbors will think that I'm a lunatic.

I'm torn between which is more upsetting to me—my uncle lying dead on the floor or having to take my mother home to sleep at our house. Just then I hear his European-accented voice. "Roberta, I'm here, I'm here." He opens the door, pulling up his pants, and says apologetically, "I was in the bathroom." Guilt attack! I'm so crazy and selfish, I dragged this eighty-five-year-old man out of the bathroom because I'm so afraid I'll have to take my mother back to my apartment.

Morris gives me the keys and I return to Richard in the car. I find myself thinking that he should have been worrying that I was raped and/or murdered because I was gone so long. But he isn't. It reminds me of when I was in primary school. I delivered prescriptions for Perlman's drugstore on Sundays. I sat in the chair next to the phone. When calls for deliveries came in, I walked to various parts of the neighborhood making deliveries. I wished my mother worried about me—but she did not. She never directed me not to go into someone's house or not to go to certain parts of the neighborhood. She didn't worry about me—and neither did Richard.

With my silent disappointment, Richard and I head back to the hospital. I've got the keys. I just need to get my mother out of the emergency room.

AFTER READING this anecdote, you may see me as a selfish and unsympathetic person. Perhaps you feel critical of me for feeling imposed upon and angry at having to take care of my elderly mother. You may feel I'm a bad daughter. Several friends read this story and said: "If I didn't know you, I wouldn't feel sympathetic toward you." The expectation that we should love our parents and not feel angry and resentful toward them when they are old makes coping with our ambivalent feelings toward them more difficult. It's painful to feel anger and guilt toward our elderly parents, but what makes it worse is the injunction to be silent. Victoria Secunda calls this injunction the "Bad Mommy Taboo."[1]

Social arrangements, like there being no public provision for the care of the elderly, induce a range of feelings, and "feeling rules" are one way that society exerts control over our feelings. Feeling rules define what we *should* feel in a particular circumstance; they serve a social function by shaping our subjective experience as it is evoked in different spheres—like taking care of elderly parents. Our culture protects the image of the Good Mother—especially when she is old. In many parts of the country and among certain cultural groups, the admission that you don't love your mother or don't like her is met with a cold stare or a gasp of horror. We are supposed to *want* to take care of our parents when they get old—it's not enough that *we do it*. We are supposed to do it because we *love* them. We can't help it if we break these feeling rules because we can't control what we *feel*, we can only control what we *do*. Yet, we feel guilty if our feelings don't fit the rules.[2]

Feeling guilty adds to the stress of middle-aged caregiving—a stage of life that many of us are confronting, but for which most of us are unprepared. My mother and Uncle Morris are part of the fastest growing segment of the population, people eighty-five years of age and older. While the total population increased by 13.2 percent from 1990 to 2000, the population over eighty-five increased 38 percent.

Half of those who are eighty-five or older need help carrying out at least one activity of daily living such as eating, bathing, going to the bathroom, dressing or getting in and out of bed. More than one-third of them depend on an adult child for this assistance.[3]

Medical advances have transformed many acute illnesses into chronic ones. Between 1990 and 2000 there was a 35 percent increase in centenarians (people one hundred years old or older). The increase in life expectancy means that elders will require care over a longer period of time and the decline in fertility means that adult children will have fewer siblings to depend upon when elderly parents need care. In addition, there is a trend toward deinstitutionalization of all but the most medically needy—the percentage of people eighty-five years or older living in nursing homes declined from 24.5 percent in 1990 to 18.2 percent in 2000. More elderly people requiring help are remaining in the community.

With so many of our parents living so long, middle-aged caregiving can last into *our* old age: Seventy-year-olds are caring for their ninety-year-old parents. In addition to all of the practical difficulties that middle-aged caregivers face, often the most painful part of caregiving is the reemergence of feelings from our childhood that seem to erupt inappropriately and make us feel out of control. The past intrudes on our experience of today. Many social workers and counselors who work with caregivers tell them not to think about the past—just deal with today. In this book I argue that we *must* think about the past to deal with the conflicts we feel and in order to do the psychological work necessary when confronted with this awesome burden.

For example, Richard and I could have had a sandwich before rushing to the hospital. But no matter how hungry I was, how could I eat when my mother might have had a heart attack? I would be breaking the "feeling rules." The adult part of me knows that things go very slowly in the emergency room and there was no need to rush—she would certainly still be there when we arrived. If we had dinner before going, I would have felt calmer and less angry. I responded in a way that *made* me feel deprived and angry—exactly how I felt as a child.

MEMORIES OF MY CHILDHOOD THAT INTRUDE

My mother never kissed me; she never put her arms around me and hugged me or told me she loved me. I often say to my sons when I hug or kiss them: "Do you know I love you?" I often ponder that. It's curious. Why isn't it enough for me to say: "I love you"? I think it's because it's so important to me that they *feel* it—because I never did. I never remember my mother holding my hand, although she must have when we crossed the street. When the other kids all ran after "Pop," the ice cream man, pushing his cart down our block in Brooklyn on warm summer evenings in the 1950s, my mother wouldn't give me the money to buy ice cream. She made a point of telling me it wasn't because she couldn't afford it (which was often true), but rather she would say: "You don't need it!" I could have tolerated not having ice cream like the other kids if the news came with a hug and the reality that money was tight for us. But instead, I felt that I was bad for wanting it—*wanting* was bad. I felt guilty for wanting and angry at her for making me feel guilty.

My childhood was spent in fear of her, hiding from her, avoiding her critical gaze. When I was still wetting my bed at ten and eleven, I never went to her in my distress. I knew she'd yell at me and announce disgustedly in front of my older sister and brother that I had wet the bed. I remember getting up in the middle of the night, after one of my repetitious dreams of sitting on the toilet and urinating. I stripped the bed, changed the sheets and mattress pad and hid them under the bed until she went to work the next day. All this I did behind her back—in terror. Each time I was sent to the store to shop for food because my mother was working, I knew I was in danger. It seemed inevitable that the A&P would have the right brand in the wrong size and the right size in the wrong brand. I would be faced with a Solomonic dilemma. I knew that when she came home from work, tired and frazzled, she would yell at me either way.

Much of my childhood was a series of similar dilemmas— trying to figure out how to avoid my mother's slaps across my face or her screaming reproaches. I didn't dust right or vacuum right or cook right or shop right. I never felt anything I did was right, so I was always trying to cover up and hide so she wouldn't find out. Sometimes I still wake up in the middle of the night, as I used to then, fearing that there is something I've done wrong, but I'm not sure what it is. There's always something. Part of me is still involved in trying (and failing) to *earn* her love.

I started planning my getaway when I was in the seventh grade. I got a job delivering sandwiches and coffee to the hordes of Jewish women who had their hair done every Saturday. No Jewish women had gray hair in Brooklyn in the 1950s; they were blonds, brunettes with blond streaks, and redheads. They spent all day Saturday reading magazines under big metal dryers with dye and rollers in their hair. I brought them coffee and bagels when they came in; I brought their lunch; and I brought them cigarettes. I saved my money in a bank account that I opened when banks offered free gifts, such as cheap cameras, if you opened an account with $25. I had accounts all over Brooklyn and I would visit the banks on my bike. I used the camera to take pictures of automobile accidents, children who got run over and other "news" that I would call in to the *Daily News*. I would get a check for my "reporting." I saved every penny and dreamed about going to college and getting away from my mother.

But after a lifetime of being angry at my mother for not taking care of me, I find myself in a position for which I am not prepared—having to take care of *her*. Despite the popular misconception that formal institutions have replaced the family as the main source of care for the elderly, in reality families provide 80 to 90 percent of the care of the elderly living in the community.[4] My view is that caring for an elderly family member is a new stage of life.[5] Of course people have always taken care of elderly or infirm parents. However, now there is a very large generation (the baby boomers) who are facing the same task simultaneously. Additionally, it is usually done for an extensive period of time because of the increase in life expectancy. Nearly half of all caregivers assist between one and four years; 20 percent provide care for five years or more.

The period spent caring for an elderly parent is not just a stage of life—it is a developmental stage because it is an opportunity for continuing the process of separation and further consolidating our sense of self.[6] During the years of our parents' decline we have yet another opportunity to integrate our parents' experience of themselves and us with our sense of self in relation to them. We have another opportunity to connect with our parents in a deeper or, sometimes, even new way.

For many caregivers it is that opportunity that motivates them. In some cases the caregiver is able to experience growth through working out unresolved feelings from childhood with the accompanying feelings of remorse, sadness and loss. In other cases the caregiver is stuck repeating the same dynamics that were so painful in childhood. I am going through this developmental stage now. I am *once again* dealing with: feelings about my brother getting special dispensations because he is a boy; my wish to have my mother appreciate me; and feeling angry at my mother for being so needy and wanting me to take care of her.

But not every middle-aged person with elderly parents becomes a caregiver. Some siblings end up the primary caregivers while others do not. Certainly, factors such as geographic proximity and employment are important. Social class and ethnic group play an important part in whether elderly parents are invited to live with their children or caregiving takes the form of paid homecare, assisted living or nursing home care. However, my purpose is to understand how family dynamics from childhood, often related to gender expectations, affect who becomes the primary caregiver in a family and how that caregiver feels about their position in the family and their relationship with the elderly parent(s).

In my case, I am the youngest of three siblings. My sister is eight years older and my brother is four years older than I am.

I was not my mother's favorite. On the contrary, I have always known that I was not a planned pregnancy. In addition, it seems that my parents wished for a Robert, but got me instead—hence I am Roberta. Clearly, my role as primary caregiver for my mother is not a result of having been her special child. My brother was the clear favorite in the family. My father attended his Saturday baseball games while my sister and I were left to clean the house under my mother's critical eye.

Since my brother was never expected to do the domestic chores that my sister and I were forced to do, he has no sense that he should be an equal participant in caring for my mother other than financially. Several years ago, I brought up the unequal distribution of caregiving responsibility between us, my brother responded: "Well, you're her daughters!" My sister seems to concur with him. She does not seem to have the same expectations of a brother as a sister.

Since women are more likely to do the hands-on nurturing of caregiving, as a dependent parent's need for assistance progresses from a need for practical help to a need for more personal care, daughters are more likely to move into a primary role.

My sister, on the other hand, has had her hands full because her husband has been seriously ill and for several years she was the primary caregiver to our elderly uncle, who was particularly kind to her at crucial and difficult moments in her life. I did not feel a similar obligation to him because he was not equally kind to me. My sister also feels that she was compelled to be "the good daughter" for many years when I was not similarly compelled. Thus, she feels it is my turn to take over. Ironically, then, I am left with the primary responsibility for my mother.

Whatever the pragmatic difficulties of caregiving, it's the interpersonal and intrapsychic factors that take the highest toll. Bonnie Walson, executive director of Heritage Day Health Centers in Columbus, Ohio, told me: "When people are involved in the acute level of caregiving, it is a huge amount of *emotional* as well as practical work. They feel like they no longer have their own lives."

I have seen many of my patients, friends and interviewees relive childhood experiences when they care for their elderly parents. My usually mild-mannered friend Carl, a specialist in pain management, was telling me about his difficulty in getting his parents to accept the help he is trying to provide for them. Finally, he burst out with: "Goddamn it, when I was a senior in college I drove my father to Alcoholics Anonymous every day for thirty days and at the end of it *he called me up drunk.*"

You may feel that my story and the stories of many of the caregivers I present are extreme examples. But the majority of people I have interviewed are living through extremely difficult situations with their parents and struggling to care for their parents while managing their own emotions and maintaining their own families and/or jobs. In Anna Quindlen's novel *One True Thing,* the daughter, Ellen, who returns home to care for her dying mother, says:

> Everyone makes up their little stories and then they wonder why their own lives aren't like that. It makes life so much simpler if we can get rid of all the loose ends. Ellen is such an angel, loved her mother so much she couldn't bear to see her suffer. Or, Ellen is such a witch that she walked over her mother in spikes to get what she wanted.

I can't be responsible for other people's stories. I have enough trouble making sense of my own.[7]

I have learned from years as a psychotherapist that there are always loose ends. Even people who seem very successful and well put together on the outside often have lived through and/or are living through very extreme experiences. One theme of this book is that caregiving *is* often an extreme situation that lasts a long time and dredges up our conflicts from a lifetime—with our parents, siblings, children and selves. It is a major challenge. But it offers us the opportunity to make sense of our *real* stories.

THE UNSEEN CAREGIVER

The National Family Caregivers Association (NFCA) estimates there are 25 million family caregivers in the United States.[8] More than one-half of all family caregivers are children and 77 percent of us are female.[9] As Gail Sheehy points out in *The Silent Passage,* more and more women are being put on "the daughter track," possibly for a decade or more, just as we emerge from "the mommy track."[10] Just as most women and men assume a woman will be the primary parent, we also assume that a daughter will be the primary caregiver for a parent—unless there are no daughters.

Fathers and mothers choose different solutions to the conflict between parenting and paid work. Similarly, daughters and sons also choose different solutions to the conflict between waged work and informal caregiving. Daughters are likelier to curtail labor force participation, while sons are more likely to reduce caregiving responsibilities. Daughters are more likely than sons to relinquish paid employment, reduce work hours and take time off without pay. Hence, daughters are more likely than sons to experience caregiving as stressful.[11]

Often, emotional stress is expressed physically because the caregiver is too guilty to tolerate her own anger. The NFCA members survey found that since their caregiving activities began: 27 percent reported more headaches; 24 percent reported more stomach disorders; 41 percent reported more back pain; 51 percent reported more sleeplessness; and 61 percent reported depression.[12]

The majority of American women between the ages of forty and sixty-four are employed. Current estimates are that between one-quarter and one-third of the workforce *also* takes care of an elderly parent. We have to deal with the demands of our jobs, children, spouses, friends *and our elderly parents*. At the same time as the need for caregiving is increasing, the difficulties in providing that care are multiplying. Increased numbers of women in the labor force, high levels of divorce and more geographical mobility make it more difficult for adult children to care for their elderly parents.[13]

I am one of those caregivers. I am fifty-eight. My father is dead. My mother is ninety-one. She's had a few small strokes so her short-term memory is not very consistent. Sometimes she is perfectly lucid and other times she can't remember how to use the telephone or what month or year it is. Despite her limitations, my feelings toward my mother are not entirely sympathetic because of my childhood relationship with her.

THE GOOD NEWS AND THE BAD NEWS

The caregiving experience offers both bad and good news. The bad news is that caregiving is a stressful stage of life for which most middle-aged people are unprepared. Just when you finally feel you've reached a plateau in your life—that is, your children are grown or you have attained success in your career or financial security and you have more freedom to enjoy life—you have to turn your attention to caring for your parents. When you feel you've finally separated from your parents and developed "adult" relationships with siblings, you have to reengage with them in ways that make you regress to your old and usually painful ways of relating to them. A sixty-year-old grandfather reexperiences his yearning for his ninety-year-old father's approval. A fifty-year-old woman gets enraged at her mother with Alzheimer's disease who asks her each day: "Why haven't you called me?"

But the good news is that caregiving can be a life-affirming experience. If you had a warm and loving relationship with your parents, it is an opportunity to show your appreciation of them and add a new level of reciprocity and intimacy to your relationship. On the other hand, if your relationship with your parents has been difficult, caregiving is a developmental stage that offers us another opportunity to work out some of the unresolved issues that are still lurking in us from childhood. During the years of caregiving, you can separate out your past and present and put your parents' way of relating to you in the context of their parents' way of relating to them. You can forgive yourself for being angry toward your parents for what they didn't give you by giving them what you didn't get. If your expectation of yourself as a caregiver combines empathy and reality, you can experience the pleasure of meeting your own expectations of yourself. And if you have enjoyed a warm relationship with your parents you may be in the enviable position of deepening and strengthening these bonds in the last years of your parents' lives.

In the course of interviewing caregivers, I have found people who have developed constructive ways of dealing with their complicated feelings about caring for their elderly parents. I have also found people who, in contrast, are stuck repeating patterns from the past that continue to make them feel bad about themselves. What distinguishes those who have experienced caregiving as a growth experience from those who are stuck? One crucial factor that distinguished those caregivers who were able to take advantage of the opportunity to once again grapple with unresolved issues from those who got caught in a downward spiral was their ability to set limits. We need to decide what we can reasonably do and then set limits on what we agree to do.

Of course, people need to set different limits at different points—there is no set recipe. It depends on the realities of your life, your comfort level and the degree to which you feel firmly separate. Setting limits in a healthy way involves balancing generosity and self-preservation and learning to accept what you have to offer as good enough. It sounds easy. But it isn't. As we shall see in the chapters in Part I, setting limits is one of the most difficult aspects of caregiving, but it is also one of the most important.

SETTING LIMITS AND
FEELING SEPARATE

The ability to set limits is rooted in the process of psychological separation which is at the heart of what is most difficult about caregiving. Setting limits is a behavioral reflection of feeling separate and clear about your boundaries. The process of separation reverberates throughout our lives; it is not a one-shot experience. It begins at birth with the physical separation from the mother's body and continues throughout our lives until final separation—death.[14] If we have a good-enough mother who cares for us as infants, but allows us to experience a tolerable amount of frustration, we realize that she is separate from us in a deeper way—we begin a process of psychological separation.[15] If she is clear about her own boundaries and allows us to go off and explore the world and return to her as a safe haven, we continue to develop a sense of ourselves as separate at the same time that we feel love and attachment.

Adolescence offers still another opportunity to work out this balance between attachment and separation. It is the period during which we attempt to adjust to puberty and integrate our sexuality into our sense of ourselves as well as renegotiate our relationship with our parents. During the end of the second year of life ("the terrible twos"), the child tries to make a distinction between self and non-self by saying "No." During adolescence the process of separation and developing a sense of identity takes the form of experimenting with behaviors that are "me" and "not-me"; rebelling against authority; testing the limits of authority and the self.[16]

If we become parents ourselves, we are challenged by yet another level of balancing attachment and separateness. We have to allow our children to become more and more autonomous while at the same time offering them love and support. Sarah, a publishing executive, recounted a story about how difficult it was for her to allow her daughter to be separate. A friend made a date with her eleven-year-old daughter and canceled it at the last minute. Sarah found it difficult to tolerate her daughter's disappointment. She wanted to make her feel better by calling the girl's mother and telling her to tell her daughter she can't break appointments at the last minute. She wanted to control her daughter's reality to protect her. Her husband made the point that their daughter needs to learn to deal with disappointment and learn that she can bear it. A simple hug or "I'm sorry things didn't work out" or the combination of both would express caring, but allow her daughter to feel separate and have her own feelings. .

Paradoxically, the more difficult our childhood relationships with our parents, the less likely that we were able to develop a sense of being firmly separate from them. Since each stage of separation echoes previous ones, childhood separation issues remain with us as adults. For example, Rebecca is a successful public relations executive but her feelings about herself are tied to her childhood experience of her mother's response to her. Rebecca's mother was depressed when she was a young child because Rebecca's father was hospitalized with manic-depressive disorder. Her mother was unable to respond to Rebecca's excitement about the world around her—she was withdrawn and distracted. Rebecca assumed her mother's lack of response was because *she* was not interesting enough to warrant her mother's attention. She was too young to understand that her mother's lack of interest in her was a symptom of her depression.

When Rebecca began treatment with me she told me a dream that expressed her experience of her mother. In the dream Rebecca was trying to get into a pawnshop that was locked. Inside were beautiful antiques and jewelry that she could see through the window, but the shop was closed and she couldn't gain access to any of the riches inside. Rebecca internalized an image of herself as not good enough to engage her mother and an image of her mother as full of goodies that she was withholding because Rebecca was undeserving. She had spent her life trying to be smart enough, funny enough, interesting enough to engage her mother and all of the mother substitutes in her life.

Separation involves seeing your mother as *not you* and her responses to you, if they were less than adequate, as a result of *her experiences, not of you.* Separation means acknowledging how limited *her* choices were. In Rebecca's case, she has come to appreciate how difficult it was for her mother to cope with the demands of a young child and a manic-depressive husband. From my psychoanalytic work, I know that there are several steps in the process of psychic separation and a great deal of resistance to taking them. Caregiving is a stage of life that involves balancing attachment and separateness; it is an opportunity to prepare for the final separation from our parents. As I will discuss in the chapters in Part II, it is generally more difficult for daughters to separate from their mothers than it is for sons to separate from mothers, daughters from fathers and sons from fathers. Since most children who are caregivers for elderly parents are daughters, I am using the term "daughters" instead of "children" or "daughters and sons."

Separating from your mother involves separating from an image of yourself as "bad daughter." If we are lucky and we had a "good-enough mother" who was able to help us separate, we feel good about taking care of our selves as well as those we love—we are able to feel that we are good-enough daughters. The worse our childhood relationship with our mother, the more important it is for us to preserve an image of her as a "good mother."[17] Otherwise *we are alone and we have no mother.* In the most extreme cases, the mother is consciously idealized—the child cannot allow any ambivalence for fear that the hate will completely overwhelm the love. In less extreme cases the good mother–bad daughter split may be less conscious. The daughter may be able to talk about the mother's faults, but keeps trying to get the impossible—to get mother to love her.

In order to protect "the good mother," we take on the burden of "the bad daughter." It gives us a fantasy of control—after all, if the problem is *me* then there's some hope for things getting better. I can try harder, do more and say the "right" thing. But if the problem is my mother's inability to mother, then there is no chance of getting what I need. This sets up the dynamic of repetition—trying to please mother (or mother substitutes), failing and feeling angry and hopeless and unlovable.

As long as you hold on to the image of yourself as "bad daughter," you cannot separate from your mother. I sometimes sit with patients whose mothers neglected or even abused them and I wonder: Why do you resist giving up such a painful image of yourself? And then I remember that giving it up feels like *being a child and having no mother.* Accepting that we cannot get what we want from our mother means giving up hope and facing a black hole. I try to remind my patients that they might be able to get some of it someplace else if they were not locked in this internal battle that depletes all their energy.

In order to separate from your mother you have to recognize that childhood feelings remain intact from when you were totally dependent on her. Although we are now adults with careers and perhaps husbands and children, we simultaneously live on another level of which we are not conscious unless we have been in psychotherapy. Our early relationships get internalized inside us and they are evoked in situations that are reminiscent of childhood experiences. When I saw a revival of Sam Shepard's play *True West,* I was struck with how much he was able to capture the power of regression. In the play, a son, who is a writer and has a wife and children, returns to his mother's home to finalize a business deal and finds his brother there. In the process of their interaction, the writer regresses and is soon overwhelmed by his feelings of sibling rivalry and desire for approval from his brother, who appears to be an aimless wanderer.

Many caregivers report similar regressions when they visit their elderly parents or have them move into their home. Karen, a sixty-two-year-old high school principal, feels humiliated when her eighty-year-old mother says: "You got a haircut, right?" and doesn't follow it with: "It looks good." She feels like a rebuked child. All her childhood insecurity and need for her mother's approval comes up in a rush.

As Victoria Secunda points out in *When You and Your Mother Can't Be Friends,* time may have moved on, but not childhood feelings and fears, trapped in a grown daughter's memory.[18] **You have to recognize the feelings and accept them as legitimate—we are not responsible for what was done to us as children.** We are as entitled to feel angry as we are to feel loving. Of course, this is easier said than done. There is a clear cultural mandate to put a good face on your childhood and not expose your grief and rage. Religious leaders often reinforce this cultural mandate rather than helping congregants work through and resolve difficult feelings about their parents so that they will be more able to provide caregiving.

One of my patients explains that the Roman Catholic schools she attended taught that feelings and actions are the same—angry feelings are as sinful as angry acts. It is very hard for her to accept the legitimacy of her feelings and distinguish between *feeling* angry and *doing* something harmful to another person. I point out that we do not have control over what we feel, only what we do. But, it is difficult to give ourselves permission to feel whatever we feel (without a therapist's or group's support).

You have to recognize your resistance to separating. My own experience and those of my patients and friends indicate that the process of separating from your mother is never-ending—it is a continuum of separation. Our relationships with our mothers turn up in our relationships with our spouses, friends and children—it's a matter of degree.

When a daughter cannot separate from her mother, and when she *will not* or is *unable to* examine why, her unresolved feelings turn up in all her other relationships—

what she could not get from her mother surfaces as an un-
realistic need and expectation. She becomes all want, little
give; all disappointment, little optimism; all appetite, little
confidence. And so she may, in the saddest sense, indeed
become more like her mother every day.[19]

Some people's relationships are a replica of their relationship with their mother, and they have no consciousness of
the repetition. For others, it is a never-ending process of seeing repetitions and trying to catch them before they have
gone too far. For example, my unresolved feelings about my
mother emerged the night of the hospital episode with my
mother and my uncle Morris.

When I returned to Richard waiting for me in the car after
my lengthy adventure trying to get my mother's keys from
my uncle Morris, I was disappointed that Richard wasn't
worried about me. I could have asked him to come with me
instead of sitting in the car. I was perfectly capable of climb-
ing the stairs to the third floor and ringing the bell. Instead,
I fell back into an old pool of disappointment and was
yearning unconsciously for a more involved and concerned
mother. I had displaced my feelings about my mother to
my husband by feeling upset that he wasn't more worried
about my safety. This was a vivid reminder of the importance of working through separation problems in the caregiving process.

You may experience significant others as if they were your
mother and at other times treat those same people as you
were treated as a child. This can feel good when you have
had a secure early childhood, but if you have very ambivalent feelings toward your mother, recognizing that you are

acting like her can be very painful—even loathsome. Ironically, the more you refuse to see your mother in yourself, the more you become like her. This book is an exploration of what we need to know in order to make a difficult caregiving process a positive developmental stage in our lives.

I BEGAN this book when I was fifty-four and my mother was eighty-six. In the intervening five years, I have become increasingly comfortable with my feelings about her. As she slips deeper into senile dementia, there is a blissful calm about her. She smiles when I arrive but sometimes thinks I'm her sister and other times her niece. Occasionally there are glimpses of her former angry self, but they are rare.

During these five years my understanding of my relationship with my mother has deepened through the process of coping with the intense feelings provoked by the progression of her dementia. I have become able to comfort my mother as well as myself because I have been more able to remember that it is *normal* and *okay* to feel ambivalent at times about my role. This book is not a "how-to" guide in the ordinary sense because each caregiver has to find her own level of comfort in the role. However, I hope it will offer you some of the support and insight necessary to find that niche for yourself.

Part I

THE
INTERNAL
STRUGGLE

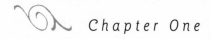 *Chapter One*

SETTING
LIMITS

When you confront an ocean of need, bring a cup.

—*The Reverend Michael Moran,*
   First Congregational Church, New Milford, Connecticut

WHEN PEOPLE CONFRONT an ocean of need they feel anxiety. Some run for their lives; others jump in and drown. Both reactions are rooted in the inability to stay separate and set limits in a healthy way that balances generosity with self-preservation. I have seen this dynamic in myself in my therapy practice and with my mother. Often, when patients feel so needy that they are desperate for me to take their neediness away, I feel overwhelmed by anxiety. I feel helpless and afraid of drowning; the feeling makes me want to withdraw. Sometimes I do, temporarily. In order to offer patients *something,* I have to be able to accept that I cannot take away their ocean of need, but I can bring a cup and offer *some* relief. I cannot do that until I am able to feel securely separate from them—clear that I am not going to drown in their neediness.

Similarly, when my mother had a series of small strokes and was increasingly unable to take care of herself, I felt overwhelmed by her neediness. She was going to a dozen different doctors who were not communicating with one another; she was losing weight and constantly complaining of nausea; she had stains on her clothes; she couldn't remember her keys or that she had just found them; she couldn't remember if she had sent her rent check or not; she couldn't remember if she had taken her medication or not; and she couldn't remember my husband's name or my birthday. She called me all the time—to ask me the same questions over and over. My sister said it was my mother's anxiety; she often felt angry toward her. My sister is the eldest child and *her* anxiety about drowning in our mother's neediness made her feel so overwhelmed that she needed to withdraw from our mother. She could hardly bear to visit her. In addition, my brother rarely visited and never indicated when he was going to. I felt guilty and frightened. What could I do? I felt that my only alternatives were doing nothing at all or letting her take me over (that is, live in my house; change my relationship with my husband and my children; interfere with my work, my friends and my routines).

I had to face a new phase in my own development. For a long time I dealt with my mother by trying to keep my distance. During high school and college I imagined whom I would go to for help if I got pregnant—my mother was definitely out. When I was in college I had mononucleosis and I was in the university hospital. I did not tell my mother. As a young married woman, I never talked to her about anything personal that mattered to me. It was easier to report on facts of my children's lives, Jason has a cold or Matthew got an A on his English paper, or day-to-day activities and events in my life, I spoke to my cousin or I went to the dentist. My withdrawal from my mother was a result of my insecure attachment to her—and that remained inside of me, sometimes consciously and sometimes unconsciously.

The early insecure attachment creates a wish to be comforted and a wish to run away from danger. The problem is that the person from whom you want comfort and the person who is dangerous is the same person—that creates an often lifelong conflict. The mother you yearn for is the mother you withdraw from; the mother you are afraid of is the mother you cling to. Children with school phobias offer a good example of this paradox—the inability to leave home is often a response to a perceived threat from the parents. Thus withdrawal and clinging are two different anxiety responses resulting from an insecure early attachment to the mother.[1]

Often, the withdrawal and clinging are split off and transferred to people other than your mother.[2] In my case, I avoided my mother, but clung to friends, lovers and my analyst. I didn't experience separation anxiety from my mother, but from my analyst and my husband.

Ever since I returned to New York from college in California at age twenty-one, I took a minimalist approach to seeing my mother. I saw her and spoke to her as little as possible. My sister enjoyed shopping with her, but I never did. I never felt good about myself in my mother's presence because I was always struggling with yearning for her to be what she could never be and being angry with her for being unable to be that. I guess what I wanted her to be was a mother with whom I could feel like a good daughter. But that was not possible.

About two years ago I realized that my mother could not take care of herself. She forgot to make entries in her checkbook, although she had been a crackerjack bookkeeper when I was a girl. She could add a long list of numbers in her head and never lose track of the total. Now she couldn't figure out where to enter the amount of the check. Her clothes were dirty and she was steadily losing weight. I had been denying it. But I couldn't deny it any longer. I had to find some way of helping my mother cope with living while maintaining my own life—bringing a cup to relieve some of her feeling of helplessness, but not drowning in her neediness.

Setting limits is difficult for most people—it's a common problem in many areas of our life, not just caregiving. It's hard to say "no" or "enough" without feeling guilty. It's difficult to tell a friend she can't borrow money or tell your son he can't have another toy he can't live without. I had a terrible time toilet training my elder son. One of my friends used to console me by saying: "Don't worry, by the time he gets married he'll be toilet trained." The more you project your own neediness onto someone else and then identify with the person to whom you are saying no, the harder it is to do it without feeling bad about yourself. I would start off feeling like a separate adult and saying: "Okay, now you're going to use the toilet." As soon as Matthew started yelling that he didn't want to use the toilet, I would start identifying with him. How can I force him to do what he doesn't want to do? I'll be acting like my mother. I'll wait until he *wants* to use the potty. Except he never got to that point. He was three years old and they wouldn't let him into nursery school in diapers so I went to a child psychologist for help. She said: "Your son does not have a problem. You do; you are not like your mother. You can tell him he is going to wear underpants and throw out his diapers and he will be fine." I followed her advice and he never had an accident again. She made it clear to me that the problem was all mine. I was so afraid of being like my mother that I couldn't set limits and stick to them. I couldn't distinguish between being sadistic and helping my son master a developmental task that would make him feel better about himself.

If we feel needy and deprived because we have an insecure internal attachment to our early mother then it is hard to say no or enough to somebody else. People who have difficulty saying no often get angry at people who ask them for anything. After all, asking them for something sets off their conflict. Thus, setting limits with needy elderly parents can be extremely difficult if we are needy ourselves—which we usually are if we had needy parents. We vacillate back and forth between identifying with their neediness and feeling we have to save them; and feeling angry at them for needing so much from us and wanting to run away so that we do not drown. Adults with a secure attachment do not feel needy— or are able to work their way out of that feeling fairly quickly. They have needs, of course, but they are not "needy." The feeling of being needy is a feeling of desperation for someone else to save you and to provide sustenance. In addition, it easily gets projected onto other people so it's hard to stay clearly separate. Caregivers who have an internal sense of secure attachment have secure boundaries and have less difficulty saying no or enough in a way that does not necessitate hitting the other person over the head with it or running away from a person who is needy. They can say: "I wish I was able to do that for you, but unfortunately I'm not."

SIBLING RIVALRY

Rose is not afraid of drowning. At forty-nine, Rose wants to be a good daughter and is angry with her mother for making her feel that she's horrible and inadequate. She wants her mother to appreciate all that she sacrifices for her.

> I'm just constantly running . . . I can't do anything right—no matter how much I do for her . . . She thinks I have nothing to do all day . . .

Rose's eighty-two-year-old mother came to live with her, her husband and two teenage children more than three years ago. Her mom had broken her hip and was discharged from the hospital after two days. Rose's brother had been living with their mom before the accident, but felt unable to care for her in her house. Medicare would have paid for her to go to a rehabilitation center to recuperate, but Rose decided to bring her home instead. After she moved in, her mom began having congestive heart failure and needed oxygen twenty-four hours a day.

When I arrived at the house to interview Rose I was ushered into a very large sunken living room. I could hear the noise of the oxygen machine from the next room, where the nurse was caring for Rose's mother. One corner of the room was taken up with the largest TV screen I have ever seen outside a theater. In each of the other three corners of the room were chairs facing the screen, rather than one another. In the

center was a huge space. I imagined people sitting in each of
the chairs having to yell to each other across the large ex-
panse of the room. Clearly this was not a room in which
people spoke to one another.

Rose told me that she has always prided herself on *not* being like her mother. She feels her mother did not set any limits for her brothers and encouraged their acting out with
alcohol and drugs.

> My brothers . . . got in trouble, they stole, and they drank.
> One of my brothers is messed up with drugs and alcohol
> every day. He just moved to Florida and came up to visit.
> It was a total disaster. He came and asked my mother for
> money and she was going to write him a check. I said,
> "Mom, that's a mistake. He'll cash the check and go to the
> bar and spend it." And that's exactly what he did.

Rose has tried not to repeat her mother's mistakes in bringing up her children.

> My brothers would come home falling-down drunk and
> she would just give them something to eat and put them to
> bed. Tell him to get out. It's called tough love.

However, in her attempt to be different than her mother, she
set so many limits on her daughters that she has difficulty allowing them to separate.

> My daughter is a great kid. I told her she has to go to the
> local community college. She had her heart set on going to
> the University of California. I said no, she has to go to

community college for one year and then she can transfer. She's never been anywhere. No, she can't go away for the first year.

Despite all her protestations, Rose is living out her child-hood script and passing it on to the next generation. Her need to be the opposite of her mother keeps her tied to her. And Rose keeps her daughters tied to her by overcontrolling them and not allowing them to develop their own inner lim-its and sense of judgment.

Using the language of Alcoholics Anonymous, Rose says her mother was an "enabler" for her father's alcoholism and irresponsibility.

> My father was an alcoholic and no matter what time he came home she got up and made his dinner and put him to sleep. He'd wake up the whole house when he came in because he was so loud when he was drunk. He spent all his money on drinking and then she worked sixteen hours a day to support us. I'm sorry, there's no way in hell that I would do that.

Rose feels bitter that her mother allowed her father's alco-holism to control the family. She resents her mother for not standing up to her father and protecting her children.

Rose has given up seeing friends, having vacations and go-ing out with her husband because her mother doesn't like it. This increases her sense of deprivation and rage. She refuses to use the $600 a month allotted to them by the state for housing her mother, which further intensifies her feeling un-appreciated and used.

There's certain things she needs and she doesn't buy them because she gives the money to everybody else [that is, to Rose's brothers]. The only thing we take out of that money is she pays for half of our electric because of the cost of the oxygen machine going twenty-four hours, the TV is on twenty-four hours, and the air conditioning is on because it takes so much energy for her to breathe that she's always hot. My electric bill is sky high.

Rose allows her mother's neediness to control her family's life. Unfortunately, Rose doesn't see the parallel with how her mother supported her father's alcoholism.

Once I tried going out for half an hour and leaving her alone. She's got Life Line. There's no reason she can't be alone for a while. Oh God! She called our neighbor and she wasn't home so she pressed the button on Life Line and the cops came. So we don't go out alone. We pack her up and take her with us.

Her mother's message was: "You cannot have a separate life from me. You have to take care of me." Her mother's tactic worked—Rose no longer goes out without her mother. Her mother never insisted her husband stop drinking or bring home his paycheck; she just organized the family around his abuse. She worked two jobs to compensate for the money he spent in bars. The family ate dinner without him; his drunken yelling awakened the children nightly. Similarly, Rose angrily accepts her mother's abuse and organizes her family's life around it.

Rose seems to think that she has protected her children

from the effects of having her mother living with them. But she can't protect her children from the effects of her feeling like an unloved child: "Sometimes I would take it out on them and I have to stop and think: 'Hey, they didn't do anything wrong.'" Rose has given up going shopping with her daughters because her mother doesn't like to be alone. She relents because she cannot tolerate her mother's displeasure. All these sacrifices increase Rose's sense of deprivation and rage at her mother.

Rose's mother did not have a separate identity herself. She sacrificed her life for her alcoholic husband and so she remains a still-dependent child at eighty-two. Never having had a mother who protected her, Rose insists on making unnecessary sacrifices for her mother/child. For example, she and her husband built her mother a huge room to live in without discussing it with her. When the room was unveiled to Grandma, she said no thanks and Rose felt unappreciated for her effort to please her mother. Despite that experience, Rose continued to try. She had her husband build a deck around the house so that her mother could sit outside, but her mother doesn't *want* to sit outside and that makes Rose feel that her mother doesn't appreciate anything she does for her.

Rose is stuck in an old pattern—trying to get her mother to appreciate her instead of taking care of her "no-good" father and brothers.

It's a guy thing. I go in and she is grumpy and nasty, but one of the boys goes in and she's all excited . . . She gets social security and a pension and it goes into her account and she writes checks to my brothers.

Rose keeps trying to get her mother to see how bad "the boys" (ages fifty-five, fifty-one and forty-eight) are. Rose is pained when they come to the house drunk and say "She's an asshole" behind her mother's back.

> The boys come here spacey and drunk and she writes them a check. Why doesn't she make my brother pay back the Visa card? He could pay $100 a month or something. She thinks I'm horrible.

When Rose complains about her brothers her mother tells her: "If you kept your damn mouth shut they wouldn't bother you." Rose feels slashed by her mother's sadism toward her, but blames her "no-good" brothers instead of her mother. Whenever she complains about her mother's sadism toward her, she immediately disavows it or blames it on her brothers.

> There's a senior center nearby and the people there have oxygen or other kinds of problems and she could spend some time there, but she wouldn't have anything to do with it. She didn't want to give me that little break. *It's not her fault that she's in this situation . . . It's not her fault that she's on oxygen. If only my brothers would help.*

Rose is caught in a tragic bind. The mother, who she desperately wanted to protect her as a child, neglected and abandoned her. Her mother always made it clear that Rose's needs were unimportant in comparison to the needs of her alcoholic father and out-of-control brothers. The insecure attachment to the person she was totally dependent upon is still central in Rose's life. She clings to the mother who still refuses to consider her needs; she feels like a little girl who cannot survive without her mother's love and protection. As Judith Viorst points out in *Necessary Losses:*

> It doesn't seem to matter what kind of mother a child has . . . or how perilous it may be to dwell in her presence . . . Separation from mother is sometimes worse than being with her when *she* is the bomb.[3]

Like so many children who had mothers who did not take good-enough care of them, she has not been able to develop as an autonomous person. Since her actions look so outwardly selfless and gallant, it's hard to see that it's not related to getting her mother the care she needs, but rather to Rose's own need to cling to her rejecting mother. Rose has no conscious understanding of her conflict. In fact, she told me that she has been having panic attacks for a few years, but she did not connect it to having her mother living in her house. She was seeing a psychotherapist to help her cope with the panic attacks, but the therapist's approach did not relate the panic attacks to Rose's early relationship with her mother. Hence, the panic attacks were getting better, but the therapy was not helping her understand why caring for her mother was so agonizing.

Professionals from an addiction/recovery background would discuss Rose's insecure attachment to her mother and consequent inability to separate in terms of codependency.[4] Rose needs to be needed. She watched her mother organize her life around the chaotic moods and needs of her father. In the language of recovery, Rose's mother was an "enabler."

Typically, codependent caregivers are, like Rose, the children of alcoholics, drug addicts, depressed or mentally ill parents.

Melody Beattie, author of *Codependent No More,* says that caregiving is a major characteristic of people who are co-dependent.[5] They feel compelled to solve other people's problems and anticipate their needs because they feel safest when they are giving. They willingly abandon their routine for somebody else because they don't expect anyone to want them for their intrinsic worth. They try to make themselves indispensable and often end up feeling unappreciated and used by others. While all caregivers have to make some sacrifices to care for their elderly parents, codependent caregivers sacrifice their happiness for others even when sac-rifice *is not required.* For example, Rose complained about be-ing exhausted, but believed she was suffering for the sake of her family. She insisted on getting up with her husband and making his breakfast at 4 a.m. despite the fact that he told her he was perfectly happy picking up coffee and a doughnut on his way to work.

My view is that what is called "codependency," in the re-covery perspective, is a set of symptoms that reflect a sepa-ration problem. Rose has not been able to separate from her mother. She still yearns for approval and recognition from her and is embroiled in an old crusade to prove that she is more deserving of her mother's love than her "bad boy" brothers. Why can't her mother see how good she is and how bad the boys are? Rose is eaten up with anger and frustration because of the unfairness of it all. On a deeper level, Rose cannot give up the battle to get her mother to mother her; she cannot face the loss of the mother she unconsciously feels she cannot survive without. Rose wants her mother to fulfill a need that was never satisfied when she was a child and for which she still yearns—the need for what psychoanalysts call "mirroring." Mirroring is the mother's smile back when the baby smiles; the smile of pleasure that comes over a mother's face when a child says something cute or does something for the first time; the mother's words of recognition when the child feels hurt or is treated unfairly. Mirroring builds up our sense of self so that we can later perform that function for ourselves. Unfortunately, Rose did not get enough of it as a child and she is still trying to get it from her elderly mother, who is incapable of giving it. She's still looking for the smile of appreciation on her mother's face to confirm that she's good.

At the same time that she desperately wants her mother's appreciation, Rose is angry with her mother for not taking care of her. But she cannot admit that directly, so she focuses on her mother's failure to take care of her sons by setting limits for them. In an attempt to give her daughters what she and her brothers did not get, she over-mothers them—which is probably experienced by her daughters not as protective as much as anxious.

Listening to my interview with Rose over and over again, I thought about what I might say to her if I had the opportunity—and I thought about how she might respond. I would try to help Rose understand how much *she* wants from her mother. Rose did not seem to be in touch with wanting anything from her mother. Indeed, she refused to use any of her mother's money to prove she didn't want anything from her. Rose finds it hard to accept that we can be grown up mothers in reality and still have feelings from when we were little girls. It's that little girl who built a big room for her mother and waited for the smile of appreciation—which still hasn't come.

ACCEPTING HIS MOTHER'S LIMITS AND SETTING HIS OWN

Paul is a sixty-two-year-old retired lawyer. He has been married for thirty-seven years and has a thirty-year-old daughter and a twenty-eight-year-old son. I met Paul's mother, Clara, at the assisted living facility where she has lived for the past two years. She is an eighty-eight-year-old woman, shrunken by severe osteoporosis, who walks with a walker. I asked several seniors at the center if they thought their children might be willing to be interviewed and Clara told me that her two daughters, sixty-eight and seventy years old, live in Florida, but she volunteered her son's phone number because he lived nearby. Paul and I met at the facility and had our first interview there. He is a paunchy man with a thick head of dark brown hair and an air of gruffness about him. As he talked, I initially felt his speech was stilted and that he was not being very open about his feelings about his mother. To my surprise, a few days later, he called me and we had a long phone conversation during which Paul expressed much more of his ambivalence toward his mother. Still unsatisfied, Paul sent me a handwritten letter clarifying some things that had come up in our two conversations. In the letter, Paul talked about the issues that were most painful to him: the time he stopped speaking to his mother and the violent relationship between his parents. Clearly, it was very important to Paul that I understand the complexity of the emotional struggle he has gone through in trying to come to peace with his ambivalent relationship with his mother.

Paul told me that his father had been a professional boxer, a proud man, a macho guy who owned a bar. He was sort of the neighborhood strongman who protected everyone. When he first bought the bar there was this gang of thugs who used to hang out there. For months he had fistfights with these guys and was taking weapons away from people. He said that his mother was a domineering woman who did not complement his father's machismo—their personalities were in total conflict. "It was like living in an arena, not a house." Paul explained that his mother had a weight problem and went to a doctor in New Jersey who gave her pills. He said that when she ran out of pills, she would lie in bed for days.

> I realized only recently that the doctor was giving her amphetamines. She became paranoid and would spy on my father. She was in a paranoid state for a lot of years.

Paul explained that his sisters moved out as soon as they could, but he was six years younger than the younger sister and was left alone to deal with his mother's drug addiction and his parents' violent relationship.

> After my older sisters moved out, my father would be away for months at a time. When he came back they would be like lovers when they first saw each other, but I knew the shoe would drop and they would get into violent fights. I would step in between them. I don't believe in men hitting women, but I don't know how he could have

avoided hitting her because my mother would get in his face and say the most awful things to him, curse at him. He would try to leave so he wouldn't hit her and she would jump in his way and not let him leave. I don't condone his hitting her, but I understand it.

His mother threw things at his father or hit him in addition to constantly cursing at him. Paul says he often thought his mother was masochistic because her behavior provoked his father to hit her.

My father was not without fault either. When things were going well and times were good, he often made stupid, inciting remarks concerning his lack of fidelity. I sometimes got the impression that he was trying to create a situation that would justify his leaving the house. They were totally incompatible from the beginning.

Then Paul gets very sad and says with deep feelings of regret:

It had a profound impact on my personality. I became the arbitrator, the peacekeeper. When I first got married, I couldn't get out of that role. When my wife had problems with how my mother treated her I would try to keep the peace. I couldn't stand up for my wife. When we had a baby, we moved into an apartment near my mother. She would stop by every day and criticize my wife; she would tell her everything she was doing wrong. My wife was respectful, but she would ask me to intercede, but I couldn't do it. It took me many years to start setting boundaries for my mother.

Social workers at the assisted living center told me that Paul is the most loving of all the caregivers who visit their parents. But he was quite matter-of-fact in describing all the things he does for his mother—the mother who never took care of his needs; the mother who provoked his father to hit her; the mother who almost destroyed his marriage.

> I try to see my mother at least twice a week. She's a very needy person. She either can't or won't do things for herself. At the beginning I tried to get her to take care of things that she could. But I have given up. I take her to doctors and dentists. I buy her things in the drugstore. I balance her checkbook and pay her bills. I used to take her to lunch a lot, but she seems more comfortable eating here.

Paul went on to describe how painful his relationship with his mother has been his entire life. He said that his mother believes that she is the center of the universe. She has trouble caring about other people. Paul feels that she tries hard to act as if she cares, but she doesn't—and she has always been this way. He told me a story about something that occurred before his mother went to an assisted living facility and that exemplifies the degree of his mother's self-centeredness.

> My mother called Friday night and my wife answered the phone and told my mother I was having chest pains and I was waiting for my doctor to call me back. My mother said to my wife: "Don't hang up, don't hang up, this is very important, you have to cancel the cleaning woman."

Clara did not express any concern about Paul having a heart attack. It was a false alarm, but Paul was hurt. Soon after that, Clara got enraged because Paul told her she couldn't sleep at his house and then she attacked his wife and daughter for not taking good enough care of her. Finally, Paul exploded and told her she was getting what she gave.

> I accused her of never really being a mother or a grandmother. I proceeded to itemize all of her abusive and neglectful behavior all the way back to my early childhood and stormed out of her house, telling her I never wanted to see or speak to her again.

She responded, in disbelief, "My God, you hate me." Paul did not speak to his mother for a year. When his sisters told him she was sick, he called her. He and his sisters decided Clara needed to be in an assisted living facility. He wanted her to move to one in Florida, where his sisters live, so they could oversee her care.

> I felt I had borne the brunt of dealing with her for so many years and welcomed a shifting of the burden to my two older sisters. Mom claimed she hated Florida and always felt sick there and refused to go.

Paul says that, at first, he undertook her care with great ambivalence. Then he realized he had to set limits on what he did for his mother.

> I spent four or five nights in the emergency room with my mother. The doctors told me she just wanted attention.

Finally I told her that she should call me from the emergency room when she was finished and I'd pick her up. She stopped calling me. If she calls and I have time, I help her. I evaluate how serious it is and decide what I will do. If I'm busy I just tell her I can't do it.

Paul set limits in other ways as well.

I let her know that I couldn't spend a lot of time with her, given her never-ending negativity. I found her very unpleasant and told her so, chastising her for her constant moaning, groaning and complaining. Over time, she has tried very hard to change, at least in my presence. She is very quick to respond favorably when I point this out to her. She has become very careful with me now. I am her only lifeline. I continually let her know I will not tolerate her unpleasantness and have, more than once, left her quickly when she became intolerable.

Setting limits with Clara has allowed Paul to feel better about her because her behavior has improved.

This has allowed for a warmer and more comfortable relationship. As a result I have spent increasingly more time with her. We have learned to make our time together more pleasant and, even at times, fun. As a result, new warmth in our relationship has emerged.

Paul understands his mother cannot feel empathy for him. He said: "Her insignificant needs are more important to her than other people's important needs." But, since his mother has been ill, he has come to terms with who she is and how she became that way.

Author Wendy Lustbader points out that the more hurtful our parents were when we were children, the more crucial it is for us to try to ascertain the wounds inflicted during their own upbringing as a way of putting our relationship with them in context. Otherwise their weaknesses become black holes into which we pointlessly pour our resentment.[6] Pouring our resentment into that black hole does not help in our healing process, but rather exacerbates the feeling of being bad. Paul has been able to feel better about himself by understanding that his mother has terrible feelings of insecurity and can't tolerate being wrong. He explained that she needs to be right and the smartest. He told me that she's so competitive that she competes with little kids to show how smart she is. He has come to appreciate her childhood miseries and how they constricted her ability to mother him.

Paul explained that his grandmother was abusive, treated his mother as a servant and clearly favored his mother's brothers over her.

My grandmother was pregnant when she was eighteen years old and had an arranged marriage to a man she never loved. It was a terrible marriage. My grandmother told my mother that her father—my grandfather—whom she loved dearly, was not her biological father. When my mother was ten, her mother kicked her father out of the house and he died when she was fourteen. She was devastated by the loss of her father. She still visits his grave twice a year, and he died almost seventy-five years ago.

Paul's grandmother took up with a man who was ten years her junior and only eight years older than his mother. His grandmother and her lover played poker day and night. Paul explains that his mother married at seventeen to get out of her mother's house, but never separated from her.

> When I was young my mother was so attached to this mother who was so hateful to her that she went to visit her in Florida when I was fourteen or fifteen and left me in the care of my sisters for the entire winter. My sisters are five and a half and eight years older than I am. When she was home, I never saw her either. She slept all day. She never gave me breakfast before I went to school or lunch to take to school. Now I realize that she was going to this Dr. Feelgood doctor in New Jersey and he was giving her speed. When she would crash she'd stay in bed all day. She forced me to go to bed early because she wanted to go out and play cards. She was never there for me.

Paul says that neither of his parents was particularly warm or loving, but he feels that whatever warmth was available was directed toward him. For example, he remembers cuddling with his parents, but his sisters say they never got that. They say he was both parents' favorite. As little nurturing as Paul got, his sisters seem to have gotten even less and hence are not eager to help him care for his mother.

Clara has not changed.

> I took her to the eye doctor's office in the city. It was hor- rible because I couldn't park. I had to leave the blinkers on and take her into the office and ride around until she was

finished and then run in and get her. It was terrible. So I found one closer and I took her there. She called me over and whispered that the other ophthalmologist's chairs were more comfortable. She has to find something to complain about. I buy her clothes and she complains and makes me return them. She calls and complains about gifts she gets. She can't accept anything gracefully.

But Paul has been able to continue to care for her by setting limits: "If she moans and groans I leave."

Paul doesn't *forgive* his mother, but he understands her within the context of her own deprivation and neglect. That allows him to take care of her in a way that is responsive to her real needs, but protects him from being overwhelmed by her neediness and his anger.

THE IMPORTANCE OF RECIPROCITY

Isabella has been able to take care of herself and her children while being a caregiver to her parents. Isabella is a forty-five-year-old mother of two sons—ages fifteen and twenty-one. She was born in the Bronx and grew up in a working-class Italian neighborhood. When she got married she and her husband were eager to get out of New York City and moved to a rural area of Connecticut. She lives in a working-class subdivision that was created from farmland. There are no beautiful old trees or flower gardens around the house—just dried grass. It is a large characterless house with plenty of living space. When Isabella ushered me into the house, I was struck by how perfectly clean and orderly it was despite the fact that she works two jobs.

When she was divorced nine years ago, she needed to work to support her two young children. She also felt that she was soon going to have to take care of her mother, who had been diagnosed with cancer, so she bought a two-family house. Her parents had a separate apartment and watched her children while she was at work. Isabella explains that the arrangement with her parents was reciprocal and there were limits built in from the beginning: "I was there for them and they were there for me. It was an exchange for the most part."

Isabella's mother died three years ago after a series of bouts with cancer. During the six years that her mother shared her house, Isabella had a lot of difficulty dealing with her.

> My mother still did that Italian Catholic guilt trip that I re-member so clearly from childhood. She'd make me feel bad if I wasn't there for her because she refused to take re-sponsibility for her own needs.

It's clear that Isabella was very angry at her mother for trying to control her and it seems that her mother used to accuse *her* of being controlling and demanding when she set limits. It seems life with mother was a perpetual power struggle with each pot calling the kettle black: "*She* was the demand-ing one . . . the controlling one . . . She tried to get me to do things *her way*. She never gave up." The emphasis on "she" implied to me that Isabella used to have trouble sorting out who was who. Was she bad for wanting to have a self, sepa-rate from her mother? Did her mother want things from her that she could not supply? Isabella had a needy mother who looked to her daughter to satisfy her needs, but during the caregiving experience Isabella began to understand, in a way she had not previously, that there are some things no one else can supply for you. She was coming to grips with her own neediness and it made her clearer about her mother's.

Isabella wants me to know that her mother did not succeed in molding her in her own image and the thought of being like her mother is disturbing.

> I have a twenty-one-year-old who lives on his own. If he calls, he calls. If he doesn't call, I call him. I don't give him a guilt trip about why he didn't call me like she did.

It seems that Isabella was able to work out some of her separation issues with her mother during the time she cared for her before she died.

> One day she said to me: "You've changed." And she was right . . . I said to her: "You're right, I'm not that person who, when you were upset with me, I'd look for any which way to make you happy because I couldn't stand you being mad at me." It wasn't that I didn't care, but I allowed her to be upset and I'd say: "Oh well."

Isabella was able to tolerate her mother being upset with her because she came to understand that her mother's wishes and her own needs were not the same. Being separate means you have to tolerate your mother's anger when your needs conflict with hers: "I grew and became so much stronger because of the connection—actually the reconnection."

Isabella must have felt very dependent and helpless as a

child, and perhaps that carried through to her marriage. But when she left her husband and had to support her children, she seems to have found a strength she didn't know she had. She was able to take care of herself and her children, and she liked that. She also liked feeling more equal to her mother, who she had always experienced as powerful and domineering. She enjoyed having her own power and not feeling dependent: "I was the breadwinner and I was the one who ran the show and we were in it together, but I was the one they counted on."

She describes her caregiving experience as a growth experience that, at times, made her angry and frustrated. But she felt that it was the best way to take care of her children, her parents and herself.

One indication that she is right in her assessment is her younger son. Bobby, fifteen years old, came home while I was interviewing Isabella. He didn't come in the front door, but entered through his grandfather's apartment. He went to say hello to Grandpa before he came upstairs to greet his mother. As he came up the stairs, before realizing I was there, he called out a warm hello to his mother. Bobby is a polite and confident teenager—very comfortable with himself. He looked me straight in the eye and shook my hand when he greeted me and came out later to say goodbye.

Part of Isabella's strength seems to come from her faith. She believes her mother is in heaven and her image of heaven seems to be a place in which people are able to come to terms with things they didn't understand in life.

When she died I knew she got it. There was no more anger and disappointment. I felt she was up there and she got it.

I knew she got what all the issues were. I couldn't get her to understand it when she was alive, but when she died I knew she got it . . . I knew she was watching from above. I was at peace and she was at peace.

Since her mother's death, Isabella's father has lived alone in the apartment downstairs. After I interviewed her, she took me downstairs to meet him. At eighty-one, he is relatively healthy. But he depends on Isabella to pay his bills, drive him to doctor appointments and shop. Isabella and Bobby have dinner with him most nights and that night he was cooking *pasta fazul.* Yet Isabella seems to be able to have a full life herself—she told me she just met a wonderful man and that she's in love.

SETTING LIMITS is not an act of selfishness, but involves caring for yourself *and* your parents. Setting healthy limits means not sacrificing personally fulfilling activities and pursuits. Feeling angry frequently is a good indicator that there is a disparity between the limits that have been set and what you need. You may be feeling angry at your parent or fighting with your spouse about your parent—either way, that's a tip-off that a renegotiation is probably in order. Rose was not able to set any limits and was chronically angry with her mother as a result.

In contrast to Rose, Paul stopped being chronically angry with his mother when he began setting limits. When she complained or said something negative about his wife or children, he told her that was unacceptable and left. Setting limits entails recognizing and accepting what you can and cannot realistically do for your parents and communicating this information to them in an empathetic and clear manner.[7]

There is no rule to follow about setting limits—each of us is comfortable with different lines in the sand. The first task is to identify your comfort level and the comfort level of your family. You may have space in your house for your mother to live with you, but that does not mean you could stand having her there—or that your husband could. The issue is not simply what you could objectively do, but also what you can emotionally tolerate. You may be happy to have your father live downstairs or close by, but not actually *in* your house. Isabella was clear that she could help her parents *and* herself by buying a two-family house and having her parents live downstairs, but not in the same apartment. She needed to retain her privacy. They were able to offer childcare and she was able to offer them emotional support and help with finances. On the other hand, you may feel good about having a parent live in your house, but not about handling the finances. There is no one-size-fits-all answer.

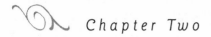 *Chapter Two*

GETTING ANGRY AND GETTING OVER IT

My father's old and helpless and I take care of him. It makes me furious that he never took care of me . . . It would be easier if I felt more loving toward him, but it all feels like obligation.

—*Joan, a fifty-year-old psychotherapist*

WHY IS FEELING ANGRY such a central part of the experience of caregivers? If you have had a predominantly positive relationship with your parents as adults, their increasing frailty or illness means you lose some of the joys and benefits of that relationship. You can no longer go shopping and out to lunch with your mother. She doesn't send a check for each of the kids on their birthdays because she can't remember the dates anymore. Your father can't pick up the kids at school or drive to your house to visit. Instead of looking to your parents for help, they need *your* help. These are real losses that may make you sad, but also angry. And you may feel guilty for being angry at those losses: Perhaps it makes you feel as if you are being selfish. You may get frightened when your mother can't remember what you told her last week. Just for a minute it feels like she's not paying attention to you and it makes you angry. Then you realize she's losing her short-term memory and it's frightening. You realize it's going to get worse and you start worrying about getting old yourself.

For example, my mother insists on walking around with hundreds of pennies in her purse. They are mixed with old cookies and bananas she takes from meals in case she gets hungry later. When I visit her I find myself getting angry because no matter how many times I clean out her purse, when I return it is heavy and smelly again. However, these twinges of anger and guilt are not the most difficult to handle. The most difficult feelings are usually related to *old* hurts and losses that get revived during the caregiving experience. This anger may feel irrational, out of control and out of place.

The cycle of anger and guilt is common among caregivers and is often related to our difficulty in setting limits. As psychologist Harriet Lerner, author of *The Dance of Anger,* points out, we often talk about the problem as if it were our parent who "makes" us angry or guilty, but no one can "make" us feel something.[1] Feeling that a parent "makes" us angry and guilty puts the responsibility on the parent to change, which is unlikely, and keeps the caregiver feeling like a helpless child. My friend Susan is caught in this bind. Susan is an attractive fifty-year-old college professor and writer who is married with two children. She writes me:

My holiday has mostly been very nice. My kids are home, which has been fun. However, my mother did manage to be hospitalized for gas. The doctor's diagnosis was: "You're full of shit!" When she called me she said: "Get me out of this hellhole. I'm dying here." Then when I arrive, "What took you so long?" That's how the day was. Two ambulances and I didn't get home until 9 p.m. She'd like me to carry her on my back.

Susan's mother feels angry that Susan will not let her live with her. Her mother does not simply want to be taken care of—she insists on being taken care of *by Susan*. Like many elderly Italian-Americans, Susan's mother expected to live with her daughter when she got elderly and infirm. Susan's mother experiences going to an assisted living facility, or even living in her own home with health-care aides, as shameful rejection.

However, having her mother live in her house would require Susan changing her life. She would not be able to wake up in the morning and work on the book she's writing; she would not be able to have dinner alone with her husband; she would not be able to have time away from her mother unless she left her house.

In my conversations with Susan it has become clear that if she moves her mother into her house she will feel continuously angry at her because her mother will not be satisfied with the level of attention and will continue to complain that Susan is not doing enough. Susan will also feel bad about herself for feeling angry and intruded upon. Her mother wants something that is not possible for Susan, but what *is* possible? Susan can talk to her mother's doctor about taking antidepressants; she can suggest counseling; she can pay an aide to pay special attention to her. But she cannot *make* her mother happy. But how can life be made tolerable for both mother and daughter?

If Susan can realize that giving up her life to try to alleviate her mother's neediness is both impossible and corrosive to her, she may be able to feel less angry toward her mother for wanting it. Susan's mother has a great deal to be unhappy about: getting old and frail; the loss of her husband; her daughter Laura's premature death of cancer; and the deaths of old friends. Unfortunately, no matter how much Susan wants to, she cannot take the losses away.

We do not, as many writers have claimed, become our parents' parents; no matter how old we are, we remain our parents' children. We may do things for them when they are elderly and infirm that we do for children (soothe them, even bathe and diaper them), but we remain their children in their minds and our own. Therefore, experiences in the present when we are adults and our parents are elderly and frail resonate with experiences from the past when we were helpless children and they were the adults we counted upon.

If we had a loving relationship to our parents and they were "good-enough" parents, it may make us angry to see them unable to take care of *themselves,* let alone *us.* We may want them to feel comfortable and happy and feel angry toward them if we can't make them comfortable and happy. That is painful. But, if we were neglected or abused as children, we may respond to our elderly parents in ways that make us feel guilty and loathsome.

For example, recently I visited my mother at the assisted living facility where she lives. She was very upset when I arrived because they had served chicken chow mein for dinner and she felt she only got a little bit of chicken and she doesn't like Chinese food. My mother told me the story in a tone of voice that was a mixture of outrage and hurt. The woman next to her, Faye, told me that you're supposed to mix up the little pieces of chicken with the noodles—it's not supposed to be a whole chicken breast. I understood completely. But my mother has always taken offense at not getting what she wants—she feels it is a personal affront. I felt angry at my mother for all the times she took offense at things that were not personal. And I felt angry at her because I often do the same thing and hate myself for it afterward. I am only able to console myself because my children will point it out to me and I see it and I apologize. Then, at least, I feel I must have given them something she didn't give me because they are able to tell me I'm being paranoid. After all that, I was able to hug my mother and tell her we'd get some chocolate ice cream for dessert and she felt much better.

When you get overly angry at an elderly parent, you need to identify the trigger that makes the anger flow and try to figure out if it is a response to something in the present or a reexperiencing of something in the past. Perhaps something in the present is upsetting, but the extremity of your reaction can be a key to realizing that something from the past is being evoked. Sometimes it is not possible to separate out past and present without getting some professional help. If your reaction is a repetition from the past, it's important to identify it before you can get over it. Some of my patients want to skip this step—they want to protect themselves from getting in touch with earlier hurts or they want to protect the parent by not getting in touch with painful childhood experiences. But, in my experience, this step cannot be skipped. It's only by knowing what hurt us and experiencing it that we can console ourselves and move on. One patient, Carla, often says: "I'm just an angry person that's all." She means that it's part of her inborn character to be angry rather than a response to experiences that hurt her. I disagree with Freud's view that aggression is an instinct. I believe anger is always a response to hurt or neglect. I tell Carla that no one is born an "angry person." She is angry because she has been hurt. Only by understanding *how* she was hurt and what it is that makes her angry can she "work through" the anger and move on.[2]

As Paul showed us in Chapter 1, understanding how our parents' experiences shaped them can be an important part of working through our anger at our parents. Whatever their history, *it does not excuse them* if they abused us or neglected us, but it helps us make sense of our own experience. Sometimes the caregiving period gives us access to our parents as people so that we are not driven to react blindly against them and repeat their hurts in our own lives—hating ourselves for what we hate in them.

Turning the furor of our reactions into a quest for understanding can be made easier if we understand our parents' histories—but it cannot replace getting in touch with the early experience. After we have experienced the hurt, understanding our parents' histories allows us to get past our fantasy that they were in control of their lives and their emotions (the angry part) or that the reason they hurt us was because we were "bad" (the guilty part).[3]

The more hurtful our parents were when we were children, the more crucial it is for us to try to understand how our parents got that way so that we can put our relationship with them in context. For example, my mother always made it clear that my father and my sister, brother and I were not her prime concern. Her first concern was getting the approval of her mother and older sister Gus. I felt angry that our feelings did not seem to matter to my mother, only what Aunt Gus or my grandmother wanted. My mother could not separate from her mother and my aunt Gus, and my grandmother could not separate from her mother either. I came to understand this when I was thirteen. My parents went to Miami Beach to celebrate their twenty-fifth wedding anniversary and I was sent to stay with my aunt Hannah, who had moved from the house next door to us, on Webster Avenue under the elevated train, to a brand-new prefabricated pastel-colored house on Long Island.

In contrast to my feelings about my aunt Gus, I loved Hannah dearly and was delighted at the prospect of spending a solid block of time with her to talk endlessly about all of the members of the family and the history of their relationships. Sure enough, Hannah and I spent the week sitting in her backyard looking at the newly planted trees and the backs of the other pastel-colored prefabs, gabbing endlessly. I was in heaven! Hannah was my mother's and Gus's older sister and the family oral historian. It was during that week that she told me a family secret that made me understand my mother in a way I never had before.

My grandmother was the eldest daughter of four siblings. I knew that. But I didn't know that my grandmother had a different father than the other three. She was born in Russia and her father was the man to whom my great-grandmother was matched—though she was deeply in love with another man. My grandmother's father drowned and her mother then married the man she loved. When Great-Grandmother had three more children with the man she loved, she clearly rejected my grandmother. Indeed, when she died she left all her money to the three children from the second marriage. If my grandmother had any doubts that her mother did not love her, her mother clarified it in her will.

So, it seems, my grandmother had a very ambivalent connection to her mother—she was overtly rejected by her. She spent her life trying to please her mother, but never could, and, in her turn, my mother grew up trying to please her mother. My grandmother asked my parents to lend her money to pay for my mother's youngest sister Mitzi's wedding. It was the money my parents had saved to put a down payment on a house; at my mother's insistence they loaned my grandmother the money. She never paid them back and they never bought a house. My mother never allowed my father to ask my grandmother to repay the loan. My mother couldn't separate from her mother. She yearned for her love and approval and my father, sister, brother and I suffered the consequences.

FINDING OUT WHAT
THE ANGER IS ABOUT

Sally is a fifty-four-year-old social work administrator and mother of two grown sons. She and her husband live in a modest house they built when they got married soon after graduating from Ohio State University. Sally is the oldest of three children. Her mother is seventy-seven and has lived alone since her husband died in 1989. Sally describes her mother as a very intelligent woman who was a history teacher. Sally says that her mother deferred to her husband in all decisions because he was very controlling, and if she did not defer, he would not speak to her for days at a time. Sally says that he used that technique on her as well: "That's probably why I became the good girl; because I had it figured out that if you were the good girl, you didn't get cut out."

When Sally's father died, her mother quickly decided to sell their house and move to Columbus, Ohio, where her three children were living. Sally says that her mother was financially comfortable and bought a condominium that had many residents her age and was close to her children and grandchildren. Nevertheless, her mother was depressed.

> There was a lot of "This isn't working out," "This isn't what I had in mind," "They don't appreciate me." She'd say to me: "You call every day, but you don't visit me—calls aren't good enough."

Sally began to experience her mother as demanding and controlling.

> She had some real health problems—she took antiseizure medication because she was having epileptic seizures; she had heart difficulties and she had stomach problems. But another way of exhibiting control is to not attend to those things, or to attend to them only partially. Then she would need intervention from us.

When Sally's mother had a valve replacement, she rejected the idea of recuperating in a long-term-care facility. She insisted that any rehab would be done in her own home. Sally, her brother and sister went along with their mother's request, feeling that it was reasonable. They knew she'd be more comfortable in her own home and believed they could arrange or provide all the care that she needed, but soon they realized that although her physical care needs were manageable, their mother's psychological needs would not be satisfied by this arrangement.

An aide came in the morning to help her mother get out of bed, get her medications in order and fix her some breakfast. Sally's brother came in the middle of the day for a visit; Sally visited in the afternoon; and her sister came before bed. There was company in attendance for most of her waking hours, but Sally's mom insisted that it wasn't enough. Her perception was that she was alone a great deal of the time.

> We started to feel angry and resentful, but how can you get angry at someone so vulnerable and frail? My sister and I thought we could fix it. We wanted to make her understand how much we were helping her, how much we wanted to help her, and that we were doing the best we could, and that we were really stressing ourselves. And after that period of time there was a long period of recovery, because she didn't believe physical therapy was necessary. So, instead of a three-month recuperation, there was a three-year recuperation, and not a return to the strength that someone of her age could have gotten.

Sally's mother's pattern of refusing to do what would help her get the care she needed and thus requiring *more* care continued when she moved permanently to Florida. She arranged, almost immediately, to have cataract surgery there, which meant she would be released from the hospital unable to see and without anyone to help her at home and no friends in the immediate area. Sally and her siblings then felt obligated to fly to Florida and stay with their mother in shifts.

Most recently Sally's mother was diagnosed with stomach cancer. After the surgery she was temporarily unable to speak or respond when spoken to. Sally had what seemed to her at the time an irrational reaction.

> That inability to respond represented to me that what I give her will never be enough, and it infuriated me. I have always, because of my relationship with my dad, avoided anger, never been honest about anger, because when you were honest about anger, it triggered his anger, and he withdrew, so you never wanted to do that. He'd shut me out, and I didn't want that to happen. So, I'm a person who can be so angry that I can't even speak, but I don't often express that in a good, healthy way.

Sally's caregiving experience brought up old feelings that she had repressed about her early experience with her mother.

> Before she had the surgery she said something very hurtful, and my thought was, It doesn't matter what I do for you, it will never be enough.

I asked her about the attention she received as a girl.

Just of not being nurtured, not being held, not being talked to the way I talk to my children. She never participated in my life as a parent. I just don't think of my mother as parenting. My mother had a friend who adored me, who would brush the hair out of my eyes. I remember her friend who had two boys holding me and loving me, and I remember sort of comparing that tactile, clear demonstration of mothering to my mother because they were friends.

I asked if she remembered her mother hugging her. She said: "No. I think she couldn't."

Sally never understood why her mother couldn't show affection to her. She didn't think about it. She went off to college at eighteen, met her husband and never lived in her parents' house again. She distanced herself and focused on her own family. But the experience of caregiving has been bringing up the feelings she has tried not to think about all these years. She never felt mothered and she felt it was because she wasn't able to make her mother happy. Sally assumed it was something about her that was the cause of it. She just accepted it unquestioningly all these years. But during a recent visit, her mother told her a story that was a psychological turning point for Sally. It explained to Sally why her mother could not love her.

Sally's grandfather was a civil engineer and her grandmother was a businesswoman at a time when being a businesswoman was a very unusual thing. They had two children, Sally's mother and her uncle John. When John was eighteen months old and Sally's mother was six years old, they were sent to an orphanage.

The children remained in the orphanage for two years and Sally's mother told her they never knew why. Although John and Sally's mother had what seemed to be a loving relationship, they weren't really close until the end of her uncle's life when they finally discussed it. It seems that each of them had been afraid to let out their feelings about being sent away, yet everything else must have seemed trivial in comparison. It must have been like trying to have a conversation with an elephant in the living room. When they did discuss it, neither of them could explain it to the other one. The mystery remains unsolved.

Nevertheless, Sally finally came to understand her mother's coldness; her mother had never been able to get over her own childhood trauma. Therefore, her mother truly wasn't there for her when she was growing up, and it wasn't because Sally herself wasn't good enough. This realization has allowed Sally to forgive in large part her mother's neediness and unresponsiveness. She says:

> How do you have a legitimate relationship, a trusting relationship with other people if you were simply sent somewhere with your baby brother? There's good reason why she would have trouble fostering a caring relationship. There's good reason why she would want to be cared for and directed.

In situations when her mother is unreasonable, Sally is able to say to herself: "Well, but it must be very hard for her. She wants to be taken care of, but she keeps setting up situations in which she feels sent away or abandoned." Being able to forgive her mother has made it less frightening to be angry with her. Sally is also more able to be direct with her mother: "We cannot take care of you if you live in Florida and we live in Columbus. We have families and jobs. If you move to Columbus, we will be able to take care of you much better." I think it might be helpful if Sally were also able to share some of her insight with her mother. She could explain to her that she cannot take care of her entirely in the way her mother wishes, but if her mother is physically close to her children she can get much more from them than if she is Florida. She can point out to her mother that moving to Florida was like sending herself to an orphanage.

Sally is using caregiving as a growth experience. She is finally understanding why she has been afraid of being angry her whole life. When her mother was unresponsive to her she turned to her father for the love and affection she could not get from her mother. But her father made it clear that she would only get his love and attention if she behaved like a "good girl" according to his rules. She understood that meant she could not show any anger.

> I've gotten to the point where I can say that I don't like the fact that you don't nurture me, that you didn't nurture me. I don't like the fact that you don't nurture other people. I don't like her very well. She's not the kind of person I would pick out. I've discovered a huge thing. I don't like my mother. I don't like her at all.

Ironically, the caregiving experience, although painful, has allowed Sally to work through her longstanding problems with anger. She has been able to get in touch with her anger toward her mother and work it through in a way that makes it tolerable—she does not have to deny it and she does not have to run away from her mother.

GETTING STUCK: HANGING ON TO ANGER FROM THE PAST

I first met Beverly in the living room of a former student of mine who is a geriatric social worker in the Bronx. Beverly is bright, psychologically minded and quite articulate. I immediately liked her and assumed she was a social worker who was going to be an informant talking about caregivers with whom she worked. I was delighted to find out that she was also a caregiver herself because I was sure that she would be articulate about her situation. She began by telling me that although she is a college graduate, she works part-time, at minimum wage, as an aide for elderly people. An only child, Beverly is fifty-five years old and single and lives with her eighty-seven-year-old mother.

> Ten years ago I lived in my own apartment and had a successful business. But my aunt and uncle who I loved dearly both had dementia and he died. I felt I had to take care of my aunt. She had no children and I loved her very, very much. She was very nonjudgmental in contrast to my parents.

Beverly experienced taking care of her aunt as an opportunity to finally have the "good mother" she always wanted (in contrast to her own mother). She rented a house for herself and her aunt and gave up her own apartment in another city.

Once Beverly relinquished her independent life because of her aunt's illness, however, she was drawn back to her own mother as well.

Before my uncle died I had pulled away from the family. But after his death, it was like, boom, I was back in the bosom of my family. All the work I had done in therapy just went down the drain. I screwed up my business. It was a jewelry business and I was doing well and then I just lost control of it.

Beverly stopped putting time and energy into her business. She stopped going on buying trips, stopped opening the store every day and stopped paying her bills. She was drawn further and further into her childhood wish to feel like a good daughter. After her father died, her mother, who is arthritic, diabetic and nearly blind, couldn't live alone.

So I decided that my aunt, the homecare person and I would move into my mother's house. So the next thing is I'm completely enmeshed in this situation. I knew when I took on my aunt that I was opening the door for my mother.

Perhaps Beverly imagined that her aunt (her "good" mother) would offset her own mother (her "bad" mother). But, instead, old resentments toward her mother suddenly surfaced with renewed force. Caregiving reactivated her childhood feelings of dependency and undermined her sense of competence and adulthood.

The first few years I lived with my mother we had some really fierce arguments. I wanted to smack her. I knew I had an enormous amount of anger there.

Beverly feels that she cannot separate from her mother until her mother dies. Her mother has to do the separating; Beverly feels she can't.

I do have the feeling that my relationship with my mother is very toxic, but I don't see myself pulling out of it. I don't see my life resuming until my mother is not here anymore. I realized last week how that pool of anger toward her is all still there and I can't pull myself out of it until she dies.

Beverly feels powerless in relation to her mother because she still feels endangered if she leaves her. Beverly's childhood feelings remain intact from when she was entirely dependent on her mother. Failing at her business and living in her mother's house intensifies her feeling that she is entirely dependent on her mother, as she was when she was a child.

She still has a lot of power over me. For example, last week my dog died. I was so upset that I didn't want to come home right after work. I wanted to wait until the vet came and took the dog away. My mother could not tolerate my feelings and my refusal to come right home. She didn't want to have to deal with the vet herself. She said, "If you do that it will be the biggest mistake of your life." And that was powerful. It took me way back. My mother

used to say that all the time when I did something she
didn't like. When my mother would say that I always felt it
was going to be the biggest mistake of my life. She always
had a power over me and she still does.

Her mother's power is based on Beverly's wish to be comforted by her and have her approval. So Beverly resists separating because she still has hopes that she will finally get
what she has always wanted from her critical mother.

I never grew up and never cut the apron strings. Am I still
trying to get my mother's approval? Probably, even though
I know I'll never get it.

Beverly understands that her mother never got her needs
met by her parents or her husband and looked to Beverly
to fulfill her wishes. Intellectually she understands that her
mother's responses to her were a result of *her own experiences.*

My mother's parents were very kissy and huggy and always
walked arm and arm and my mother felt very left out.
When she married my father, she very quickly learned that
he was in his own world and he wasn't going to give her
what she wanted. So when I was born all her hopes were
on me.

Beverly understands her mother's neediness, but she still
feels that she has to satisfy it and drown or be a bad daughter. As a young woman, she felt she had to run away to preserve her sense of self, and then yearned for a fantasized
connection with her mother. When she came back, she hated

her mother for being so critical and needy and making her feel like a bad daughter all over again. She goes back and forth between longing for her mother and having to run away out of fear of being gobbled up by her.

Before she moved out of her apartment and rented a house to share with her aunt, Beverly was in therapy. What did that therapist say to her when she told her what she was going to do? Of course, I don't know. Maybe the therapist warned her that giving up her apartment was not a good prognostic indication. She could have made sure her aunt was well taken care of and visited her frequently without giving up her apartment (and her own life). The therapist might have said that and Beverly did it anyway. She ended therapy when she moved in with her aunt and later her mother.

Beverly feels that the pool of anger toward her mother is all still there and she can't pull herself out of it until her mother dies. She feels that she cannot set herself free—only her mother has the power to set her free, by dying. Beverly explains by saying she feels she "should" take care of her until she dies. If she does not take care of her she will be a "bad daughter." However, Beverly *is* taking care of her mother and still feels like a bad daughter because she is constantly angry and guilty.

Beverly feels that no one ever asked her what she *wanted*— she was just told what she should do. She feels like she has no choice. However, the reality is that Beverly does have a choice. The choice is between continuing to feel like an angry helpless child living with her mother and hating her vs. moving out of her mother's house, hiring an aide for her and getting a job that is appropriate to her education and skills. It seems like a no-brainer. Why does Beverly opt for the self-destructive choice? There must be something that Beverly gets out of choosing to continue the sadomasochistic dynamic with her mother. Perhaps Beverly feels that this is the only way to have *any* relationship with her mother. If she gives up feeling angry and helpless in the face of her powerful and sadistic mother, what will she have? She will feel alone.

Beverly thinks that when her mother dies she will be free of her. But that's not true; she is tied to a relationship to her mother that will outlive her mother. She can move away, her mother can die but the internal relationship to her will live on. Beverly's mother will be alive and well inside Beverly when her mother is long dead, unless she is able to understand her need to hold on to being the angry, victimized, misunderstood daughter of a needy, dependent, yet powerful "mother." The image of herself vis-à-vis her mother will outlive her mother. For example, why is Beverly so underemployed? She is a highly intelligent college graduate with years of business experience, but she works as a minimum-wage health aide. She needs to remain the tortured, undervalued daughter in order to hold on to that inner relationship with her mother.

How would this understanding of her situation help Beverly? If she were aware of her own part in perpetuating this old masochistic relationship with her mother, Beverly might be more able to make choices about her life. If she saw that she *could* move out and get a job and have her own life, but that she is *choosing* not to do that, it would be harder to continue feeling like her mother's victim.

Beverly's caregiving experience caused a major regression and repetition of her early experiences with her mother. She is stuck feeling enraged at her mother and unable to work through her anger in a way that would allow her to separate from her mother and have her own life. What might happen if Beverly *did* leave? What would happen to her mother? She has money and could afford to hire aides to live in the house and care for her. She does not have the same expectations of aides that she had about Beverly. Just as Beverly's angry feelings are evoked by her mother, her mother's needy and angry feelings are evoked by Beverly. They are locked into an interaction with each other that they keep repeating. If Beverly moved out she might find she *wanted* to visit her mother and make sure she was cared for; it might feel like a choice rather than a duty she cannot escape. It is possible to use the caregiving experience in a more life-affirming way—to use it as an opportunity to work out problems that have been left unresolved or simply to resolve them more completely.

GETTING OVER THE ANGER BY SETTING LIMITS

Paula is a fifty-four-year-old round-faced woman with graying hair that's curled unevenly. She looks like a woman who cannot be bothered worrying about how she looks—her values lie elsewhere. She is a fund-raiser for a large nonprofit organization.

Although Paula has five children and works full-time, she is the caregiver for both her mother and father—they were divorced right after Paula graduated from high school so she has to deal with them entirely separately. Paula's mother is eighty-four and her father is eighty-seven. Her father is an alcoholic and twelve years ago he had surgery and got pneumonia and was incapable of living on his own. He lived with Paula and her family for six months and then they got him an apartment in an assisted living facility.

Paula's mother had a recurrence of breast cancer six years ago. She lives in independent housing, but her dementia is increasing and Paula says that the next time her mother is hospitalized, she is going to put her in a nursing home afterward. When she goes to the doctor, she cannot remember why she's there. She's safe right now, but only because Paula keeps her medication and gives it to her every day. Paula's mother goes to the senior center three days a week. But Paula is increasingly concerned about her safety the rest of the time.

Paula says she had "an abnormal childhood."

> My father was always an alcoholic and it was an elephant in the room—no one ever talked about it. My dad was home every night because my mother worked as a waitress at night. But he was not emotionally there.

Paula says she always felt like she had to be the mother. She did the shopping and cooking because her mother wasn't there and she was the eldest girl. When her parents' marriage fell apart, Paula felt that she had to be even more grown-up.

> My father was never a falling-down drunk, but when my mother left him he started to drink more heavily. She was a waitress and she had an affair. I knew it. It was very painful. My junior year in high school, I saw my mom and a man go into my aunt's apartment. I knew what was going on.

Paula's mother kept saying: "Someday you'll understand."
Paula says:

> To be candid, I never did. I don't agree with the way she
> handled the whole situation. She's not real brave. She's al-
> ways had to rely on a man. She's never had the strength to
> be on her own. She left my sister and me with my dad and
> moved in with my aunt and eventually married the man
> she had the affair with. It was very difficult.

Paula says that her mother's two sisters were very supportive
of her affair. She felt shocked by her aunts' reaction. One of
them called Paula and yelled at her for not being supportive
enough of her mother after her mother left the family. Paula
shakes her head in disbelief as she tells me about it. She doesn't
completely understand why her life is so stable considering
what she's been through. Clearly, Paula's "plain Jane" presen-
tation of self is in contrast to her mother's overt sexuality. As
a young woman, she says she was petrified that when she
got married she would want to have affairs like her mother.
She can chuckle about it now, but it's clearly taken years
for Paula to work through her feelings about her mother's
infidelities. Paula says:

> She's eighty-four years old and she's still a flirt. She's flirt-
> ing with the sixty-eight-year-old van driver who takes her
> to the senior center. She wanted to invite him over and I
> said: "Sure, let's have Earl and his wife over." She looked
> like I punctured her balloon. She was so disappointed. It's
> comical. It's also interesting. As we age we become more
> of who we are. She's a youthful and attractive eighty-four-

year-old. She has to have her hair done every week. You might go out on the weekend, you never know. My kids say: "Grandma's getting more action than we are."

Paula doesn't feel her siblings fared as well psychologically as she has. Paula says her brother was her mother's favorite child. During World War II when her father was overseas, her brother lived with his mother and aunts. He was the only child and a boy at that. When his father returned, his aunts left and his mother turned her attention to her husband. Then she got pregnant with Paula. Paula feels her brother's privileged position came to an abrupt end and he never got over it. He and her father fought constantly, so as soon as he graduated from high school, her brother joined the army and went away. He doesn't talk to either of his parents or Paula. She said he occasionally talks to their younger sister. Like his mother, he started having an affair and left his wife, a close friend of Paula's, and two children to marry his lover. Paula did not support his affair the way her aunts supported her mother's and as a result her brother doesn't talk to her.

Paula says her younger sister is in worse shape. Her mother used to openly refer to her sister as "the accident." Paula says that even as a kid she knew that was not right. Her sister got married at sixteen—no doubt to get out of the house, but she got divorced two years ago. She suffers from severe depression and has tried to kill herself twice.

Paula feels angry and resentful that she is the caregiver for both her parents. She says simply: "I feel responsible. I always have." Paula feels her sister is incapable of helping, but she feels angry toward her brother.

Knowing that I have a brother who is wealthy and could make their lives easier—they both live on social security and live in subsidized housing. They're on Medicaid assistance. I don't feel as resentful toward my sister. I am stuck.

Then Paula makes an unconscious slip. She says: "I do have other children." Obviously, she feels she has to parent her parents as well as her children.

Paula has had to struggle with her anger at her father as well as at her brother and mother. Her father's drinking makes her angry. She says:

Two years ago we went to pick up my dad to go to church on Christmas Eve. We had this tradition that everyone comes to our house for Christmas. We got to his house and he had been drinking to the point that it was obvious. I said: "We're not going to do this." He was furious that he was left alone on Christmas Eve. That was really tough.

Paula felt that she had to protect herself and her own family.

I felt guilty, I'm a Catholic, and it's terrible to leave someone alone for Christmas and Christmas Eve. But I realized that God wouldn't want me to be angry and resentful on Christmas. It's a balance. I knew I was doing the right thing for me.

Paula explains more about her father. She says her father can just "go off" on anything. He's even more difficult to be with than her mom. Paula says:

He's always complaining. He has an entitlement mentality. He never says: "Gee, it's nice to do this." Instead he says: "Why didn't you ever do this before?" It was making me nuts.

After her father moved in with her family, about thirteen years ago, Paula went into therapy because it was such a demanding experience. She was depressed. She describes her father as very authoritarian—the kind of father that hit you with a belt. She says it's hard to separate the effects of the alcohol and his personality. "We were supposed to be quiet little girls and say: 'Yes, sir' and 'Yes, ma'am.'"

Paula says therapy helped her realize the depression was about anger.

I was always that kid who wouldn't say "shit" if I had a mouthful of it. Therapy helped me accept my angry feelings and realize that I had choices and options.

The burden of caring for both her parents and trying to deal with the anger it evokes is intensified by Paula's concern about her older daughter's health. Her daughter had melanoma in three locations. Paula says, tearfully:

Here's this beautiful girl with a beautiful baby and she has cancer. I didn't tell my mom because I knew she would forget right after I told her. I would be very angry at her for casually saying: "How are the kids?" I knew my father would call her and keep asking her: "How *are* you today?" He would hound her. So I didn't tell him. My daughter goes for checkups every six months and she's okay. But dealing with the day-to-day trivial things for my parents feels more annoying when I'm thinking about my daughter.

For example, Paula's mother ends up in the emergency room all the time. She calls 911 and they send an ambulance and Paula ends up having to go there and spend hours and hours waiting until they determine that nothing is wrong.

One time, after spending eight hours in the emergency room because she decided she was bleeding internally, it turned out she had taken Pepto-Bismol and that caused the black stool.

Paula came to realize that she was either going to have to stay away from her parents, which was what her brother did, or set some boundaries.

I used to feel that every Sunday I had to have one or both of my parents over. Then I said: "Why am I doing this?" I finally decided to do it every three weeks or so. I was becoming the victim. There's a fine line in my mind between feeling angry and resentful at situations and becoming the victim. I felt that the only way not to feel like a victim and hate them was to carve out that niche for myself and say: "I will set the terms."

Paula asked herself: "Do I want to walk away like my brother?" She decided she wouldn't be able to live with herself if she did. So she has learned when to take her mother's complaints seriously and when to let things go. There are days when Paula can't get to her mother's house and she misses her medication. Paula has learned to accept that it won't kill her mother. She is able to keep her priorities very clear.

TO VARYING DEGREES, Beverly, Sally and Paula were able to work through their anger at their mothers (and for Paula, her father as well). While Sally and Paula were able to get in touch with their feelings, accept them and then move on, Beverly remained stuck.

Both Beverly and Sally felt they were bad children. Beverly was very aware of the feeling her whole life, but Sally didn't realize she felt it until she started to care for her mother and got in touch with it. Ironically, the child who has a "bad" mother usually turns her into a "good" mother. That necessitates feeling that you're a "bad" child. That does not feel good, but this defensive process that defines as "good" the person you are dependent on serves an important psychological function for a child who needs that mother. If the child can turn to the father or grandmother or older sibling, she may be able to tolerate more ambivalence toward her mother, but if there is no one else to turn to, the child may prefer to feel that *she* is bad, not Mommy. I have seen this in many of my patients. The alternative is to feel your mommy is bad and you are helpless, alone and orphaned. Sometimes the feeling alternates—"I hate Mommy" and "I'm bad." However, the process that might have served them well as a child becomes an impediment to feeling good about themselves as adults.

Beverly's situation was, and is, more dire than Sally's. Although she was fond of her aunt and uncle they did not play a large role in her day-to-day life. She was dependent on her mother as a child and still is as an adult. At fifty-five, Beverly is still hating her mother and hating herself.

On the other hand, Sally was able to turn to her father for love when her mother was unresponsive to her as a child. That allowed her to feel more ambivalent about her mother, and she did not have to defend against her negative feelings toward her mother by feeling like a bad daughter; she just had to be a "good girl" to keep Daddy's love. Caring for her mother allowed Sally to understand her relationship to her mother and father much better. It freed her so that she could stop being a good girl and become a mature woman.

Similarly, caring for both her parents allowed Paula to stop being a good girl as well. She realized that she would have to set limits with both her parents in order to protect herself from feeling like a victim and to protect them from her need to run away.

Chapter Three

FEELING GUILTY AND FORGIVING YOURSELF

> I'm forty-one and have been the caregiver to my mother for the past thirty-one years. I have some nursing help during the day so I can keep my job, but I'm at my limit. I had to refuse better jobs because they're too far away for me to dash home if there's a problem. I'm on medication for nerves and depression and my own health is suffering. I've pretty much decided that it's time to call it quits and place my mom in a nursing facility. But she wants to die at home and I cannot honor her request. I am sure she will use every guilt tactic in the world. How can I deal with the guilt that comes with saying: "I give up and I have to disappoint my mom."[1]

AS CAREGIVERS, we often feel guilty for not rescuing our parents from the pain and discomfort of old age. But we cannot rescue them; we can only offer our love and support and hope they accept it. Yet, many of us *do* offer that to our elderly parents and *still* feel guilty. What is this guilt about?

In my experience and in my discussions with other caregivers I have found a variety of complex experiences that we refer to as "guilt." Some forms of guilt have to do with not meeting other people's expectations, while other forms have to do with not meeting our own.

There is the guilt we feel when we don't do things that we think we should. These "shoulds" are injunctions that we have not completely internalized as our own. When you say, "I should visit my mother every day," it really means you imagine someone else thinks you "should." Perhaps you imagine your relatives think you should visit your mother every day.

When you think, "I should make dinner for my family instead of visiting my mother after work," you are not saying you think that's right or that's what you wish to do. Rather, you are expressing the feeling that other people, perhaps your husband, thinks that's the right thing to do. Conflicting "shoulds" can be quite anxiety provoking, making you feel torn in many directions.

Then there is separation guilt—the guilt that communicates: "I am a separate person, I have different values or different needs than you do. We are not one." Separation guilt may emerge as a result of physically separating from your parent, moving to a different city, for example. But separation can be symbolic as well as physical. Making different choices about how to live your life can give rise to separation guilt as well. Each move toward self-development can feel like betrayal of your mother because you are living your own separate life.

And there is guilt as a result of having an envious mother. One of my patients feels guilty for having anything more than her mother. Her mother did not enjoy her daughter's achievements; she was contemptuous of them because she was envious. Having sensed her mother's envy beneath the contempt, my patient feels guilty for going to graduate school when her mother left school after high school to care for her sick father. My patient finally admitted she was even guilty for not having arthritis and cancer as her mother did.

On the other hand, there is moral guilt—a response to a violation of our own moral code. If you've spent your life believing elderly people should be kept in the community and decide to put your father in a nursing home, the guilt you experience is "moral guilt." Moral guilt is painful because it shakes your sense of self and involves a reconsideration of beliefs you took for granted.

There is also the guilt that one experiences as a result of ambivalent feelings toward a parent. If you are angry toward your mother when you have to decide whether to put her in a nursing home, there is always the question of whether you are doing what your mother needs or if you are trying to hurt her.

And then there is the guilt of feeling you are the special one who can offer comfort and solace, but other exigencies of your life (like living far away) make you unavailable to do so. Sometimes it is true that you are the only one who can offer comfort and solace, perhaps you're an only child and your parent is widowed. That is a painful conflict when you have other obligations that are equally compelling—young children or a sick husband. However, in some cases feeling that you are the only one who can offer comfort is *a wish to be special* rather than reality. In that case, as painful as the guilt is, it is the price for feeling special. Feeling less guilty involves the realization that you are not the only person who can provide some comfort for your mother, allowing you to mobilize other people to do so.

Although I have tried to delineate various types of guilt, we usually experience more than one type at the same time and the common thread among them is that they all make us feel bad about ourselves. When psychoanalysts talk about guilt they are usually referring to "neurotic guilt"—a feeling about a wish or fantasy rather than an action that caused damage to another person. According to Freud, the neurotic sense of guilt arises as a result of conflict between the superego, an internalized set of expectations, and infantile sexual or aggressive wishes. While the types of "guilt" I have discussed go beyond what Freud was talking about, they all involve turning aggression inward.

My friend Susan suffers from "shoulds" and from separation guilt. Susan's mother was born in Italy and feels that daughters are obligated to have their parents live with them when they get old. She feels angry that Susan will not let her live with her and Susan feels guilty. Susan feels she "should" invite her mother and if she were a good daughter she would. But Susan was not born in Italy. She is an American-born writer with a Ph.D., and she does not believe that daughters are obligated to have their parents live with them; she just feels like she "should." In addition, Susan suffers from separation guilt. When she says, "No, you can't live with me," to her mother, she is also saying, "I am a separate person, Mom, I have different values from yours. I don't want to live my life the way you did."

What might help Susan allay her guilt and forgive herself? She has to think about whether she agrees with those shoulds. Who is it that thinks she should do this or that? What does she believe is right? If what she believes is right does not coincide with the shoulds, then she has to decide if she wants to mold her life around what others think she should do. Susan knows that if her mother moves into her house she will feel perpetually angry toward her because her mother will not be satisfied with the level of Susan's attentiveness to her. Susan will also feel bad about herself for feeling angry toward her mother for intruding in her life and violating her privacy. Her mother wants something that Susan does not want to give. Susan has set a limit.

If Susan cannot give her mother all that she wants, what *can* she do for her? She can fulfill her own moral standard by finding a warm, safe environment for her mother where she will have social contacts and be taken care of. She can talk to her mother's doctor about prescribing antidepressants. But she cannot *rescue* her mother. She will only drown trying.

THE BURDEN OF TRYING
TO SAVE YOUR MOTHER

Sharon is a forty-three-year-old social worker for the New York Department of the Aging. When I met Sharon at the entrance to the senior center, she seemed rather cold. I was surprised because a mutual friend told me that she would be happy to talk to me. However, as soon as I closed the door of the interview room I realized why she had been cool when shaking my hand. She was trying to control a flood of emotion—she started to cry as soon as she sat down to talk about her mother.

Sharon explained that her mother had died about six months ago. Her guilt was evident immediately.

> I couldn't be there every day. She was far away in another state. She and my father moved to Pennsylvania in 1993 to be closer to my sister.

Sharon feels that she "should" have been there every day, even though her mother lived in another state and her sister lived nearby.

Sharon is the youngest of four children. Her eldest sister died four years ago of breast cancer at fifty-two. Her brother is nine years older and another sister is four years older. Her surviving sister, Joan, lives in Pennsylvania and her parents moved there to be near her and her two boys. Sharon's father died suddenly two years ago and her mother began sliding downhill. She had heart problems for many years and became more and more isolated after her husband died.

> It became more difficult for Joan to spend time with Mom. When Dad was alive they used to go to the boys' games and things like that. But Mom wasn't interested in those things herself and it was hard for Joan to take time out from work, commuting and her kids to spend time with Mom separately.

Sharon's mother was too high functioning to be in assisted living and the only senior center was far enough away that she'd have to drive there, but she couldn't do it and Joan could not take her mother there and pick her up. Sharon is conflicted about her sister Joan. On the one hand, she is protective of Joan—she made it clear to me that the limited attention Joan could offer her mother was perfectly understandable: "She called her every morning." On the other hand, Sharon seems to feel that Joan invited her parents to move close to her (which was farther from Sharon than their original family home) for selfish reasons and did not intend to take responsibility for their care.

> My sister made a commitment to my parents when they moved near her, but she didn't think about what it would be like when one of them was gone. When my father was there it was fine. He played with her kids and went to their ball games.

One morning Joan called her mother and there was no answer. When she rushed to her house, she found that her mother couldn't get out of bed. She couldn't move; she had a severe kidney infection and it caused terrible back pain. Soon after her mother was hospitalized she became depressed and Sharon, who feels particularly responsible for making decisions about her mother's care, decided to ask her mother's doctor to prescribe antidepressants. Her mother came home from the hospital and stayed with Joan for a few days and then went back to her condominium. Sharon went down to stay with her and talked to her about assisted living.

Sharon soon found a beautiful assisted living facility with different levels of care for her mother and she was doing pretty well. Sharon drove from New York to Pennsylvania to visit her every few weeks and stayed several days each time.

Then her mother had two falls; she was having some issues with balance and it wasn't clear why. Sharon got her mother a walker and thought that was really positive, but then her mother started showing signs of Alzheimer's disease.

I had done all this research on Aricept [the memory-enhancing drug for Alzheimer's patients]. Here in New York people think it's a wonderful drug, but in Pennsylvania they don't think that. My sister's personal physician did not feel very good about it. I called all the specialists I know and they all thought it was good and so I pushed for trying it. I thought it would help to get her back on her feet so she could adjust to assisted living.

Sharon was sobbing when she explained that her mother got up in the middle of the night, climbed over the bed's protective bar, only to fall and smash her pelvis. The physician said it was so severe she'd never walk again. Sharon's mother became increasingly confused and lost more and more weight. At this point in the interview, Sharon was crying so hard that she could hardly speak. Sharon is clinically depressed as a result of her guilt. She feels that she should have known that Aricept could cause dizziness. She imagines people must think she's a terrible social worker because she made that decision.

I feel very guilty that I didn't just take off and stay with her for six weeks until she was in good enough shape to move into her apartment and also that I was the one who pushed for her taking Aricept. My sister looked to me to make these decisions because I'm the professional in the field. If

I had lived there or I had taken her home to live with me it wouldn't have happened. I *could* have done that.

At this point in the interview I was struck by Sharon's feeling that she could have saved her mother. I pointed out to her that she seems to blame herself for something she could not have possibly known. After all, she had spent a lot of time and energy finding her mother an appropriate place to recuperate and researching the pros and cons of Aricept.

After the fall, I was so miserable. I couldn't sleep. I was going to bring her up here. But then my sister would have a hard time coming up here and my brother could see her more easily in Pennsylvania and my mother's one and only brother lives in Baltimore. It would be much easier for him to get to Pennsylvania than New York. I decided it would be selfish to bring her here. I visited her as much as I could.

I remarked to Sharon that she seemed to feel *she* had to take care of her mother, but do it in a way that would be convenient for everyone else. She seemed to be making excuses for everyone else and didn't consider her own needs at all. Then she explained:

My mother had a long history of heart problems. Throughout my childhood I lived in tremendous fear that my mother would die. My mother worked in a factory and she was often taken out of the factory by ambulance. She worked three shifts and there were lots of times she wasn't home for dinner and my Dad and I would fend for ourselves.

Although Sharon is a social worker and does counseling, she seemed to be completely oblivious to how that childhood experience of being terrified her mother would die had affected her. She did not realize the connection between that childhood experience and how responsible she felt for caring for her mother. The little girl in her was desperate to keep her mother alive.

> I never anticipated that my mother's illness and death would do this to me. As a child I was a caregiver. I knew even when I was a kid that I wanted to be a social worker and help old people. She'd come home from the hospital and I'd cook and take care of her. Every time my mother got sick as an adult and went to the hospital, my father would call me. It's really the only time my father would call me.

Sharon feels like a failure because her mother died. She failed at her raison d'être—saving her mother.

> My sister has none of these feelings. I think she wasn't the caregiver that she could have been, but she doesn't feel guilty. My brother has never been involved in my parents' lives. He doesn't feel guilty. My sister did not see sacrificing to care for my mother as an obligation. I would never have asked my teenage boys if Grandma could move in like Joan did. They said no. I would have told them she's moving in.

Sharon knows that she felt responsible for her mother in a way her sister and brother did not. But she does not understand that it is a result of having spent her childhood feeling responsible for keeping her mother alive. That is a huge responsibility for a child; it is both a terrible burden and a special position of power. Sharon's sense of self was built around being a powerful caregiver—perhaps that had something to do with her choice of profession.

Sharon feels that as an expert in her field she should have been able to save her mother. However, I view the situation differently. Sharon's sense of being able to take care of other people was based on her feeling of potency from caring for her mother. Being unable to save her mother strikes at the heart of Sharon's sense of self. She has not only lost her mother, but her image of herself. Sadly, Sharon told me that for the last six months she's been wondering about whether she wants to leave the field of gerontology: "I'm a professional. This is what I do. I should have done the best job for my mother."

She also suffers from separation guilt. She did not bring her mother to live with her, nor did she leave her job and move in with her. She had a separate life and continued to live it. That makes Sharon feel guilty. If she were a "good daughter" she feels she would have given up her life to care for her mother. Finally, she is guilty because she feels she did not live up to her own moral values.

I have been so against institutions all of my life. It's such a value to me. I never should have let her leave home. I should have gotten live-in help for her.

ANGER AND GUILT

Sara is a forty-six-year-old university administrator. She and her husband live in a nineteenth-century building in one of Manhattan's most beautiful neighborhoods. Ringing the bell, I admired the beautiful wood door in the entry area. I loved the mahogany in the halls and the beautiful moldings. When she greeted me at the door, Sara seemed much more relaxed than when I had called her to set up our interview.

As I gushed about the beautiful apartment, Sara explained that her husband, Chuck, bought it five years ago—just before they met. Most of the furniture was his—the large burled mahogany coffee table and matching end tables, the dining room table and chairs. As we settled down to talk, I sank into the couch facing Chuck's extensive pottery collection while Sara sat in a chair facing me.

While Chuck was married before and has children, Sara never lived with anyone before Chuck. She has spent much of her adult life caring for her parents. After a long illness, her father died two years ago and her mother passed away a little more than a year later. In those last two years, Sara had to make life or death decisions for both parents. Interestingly, she feels little guilt about removing her father's respirator, but has not been able to resolve the guilt she feels about not putting in a feeding tube for her mother.

Sara's father worked until he was seventy-nine and needed bypass surgery. He never fully recuperated from that surgery. The nursing staff did not make him get out of bed and walk around. He didn't get any exercise while he was in the hospital. He got an infection while he was in the hospital as well.

He went downhill over a period of two years. He was hospitalized four times and went into rehabilitation each time, but ended up losing his foot. He never went back to work.

At the same time her father was in the hospital, Sara's mother was in the early stages of Alzheimer's disease.

He couldn't really go back to their apartment and have my mother care for him, but I didn't realize that. In fact, he may have gotten the infection that caused him to have his foot amputated because of poor homecare. She would leave the apartment for hours and we didn't know where she was.

Her father went back to the hospital and then to a rehabilitation hospital. Sara says:

I ended up going to visit my mother at the apartment and then to the rehab hospital to visit my father. But I didn't know where my mother was sometimes. She would wander onto the highway. I called every hour. I didn't know where she was. I was a wreck. She wouldn't accept any homecare. Her house smelled like feces and the refrigerator was full of rotten food.

Finally, Sara knew she had to get help for her mother. She contacted a homecare agency, interviewed various aides and chose one.

I took the day off to take her to my mother's house. They spent time together alone and I also watched them interact and I hired the woman. As soon as I got home there were two phone messages from the agency and two from my mother. She took this woman's things, threw them into the hallway and locked her out of the house.

Sara was intensely frustrated. She knew her mother needed help, but she would not accept it. She got a geriatrician to do a home visit and he suggested giving her a tranquilizer that would calm her down so that she would accept help. He said she had Alzheimer's and that people with cases less severe than hers were institutionalized. He said she couldn't be left alone. She either needed homecare or a nursing home.

I thought she'd be happier at home and my father would be coming home soon. She loved the doctor and I explained the pills to her and then I went home and called her and asked her about the pills and she said, "What pills?" She had taken all of them. I realized I needed to institutionalize her.

Sara had to make the decision to send her mother to a nursing home while her father was in the ICU on a respirator. Making the decision alone was very difficult. Sara was concerned about how to get her mother to go. The geriatrician said she should tell her she had an appointment with her regular doctor, whose office was across the street from the nursing home. He suggested that the doctor would then give her mother a sedative so that Sara could take her across the street to the nursing home.

One of the hardest memories was her dressing up to go to the doctor's office. When I was taking her to the nursing home I knew it was the last time she would be in her house. It was terrible. I got her to the doctor's office and he was really unprepared. He didn't have the medication that was going to make it easy to get her over there. I had to go to the pharmacy to get the drugs. She had to sit in the office and wait and the other patients were complaining that she smelled.

In the Alzheimer's unit in the nursing home, she was sometimes aware of what was going on around her—that was painful for Sara to witness. Then there were times her mother would slip into oblivion and needed the services that were available. She kept trying to find ways to get out.

When I was leaving her in the nursing home she was chasing after me: "Don't leave me here! Don't leave me here!" It would have been a hard thing to do if I really felt loving toward my mother, but it was even worse because I didn't.

Sara was wracked with guilt and anger. She knew her mother had to stay in the facility but felt guilty because she wanted to leave her there. She wanted someone else to care for her.

Sara had good reason to be angry with her father as well, but she was more able to express her feelings to him and be heard toward the end of his life. She explained that when her father moved from her childhood house to an apartment in the city, she went there and packed up the things that were most important to her and put them aside in a box. Her father, after forty-six years of living there, just threw everything away. When she went to get the box it was gone. Sara says:

I was deeply hurt. These were the things that were most important in my life. All my toe shoes were in the box. He didn't protect me. I was furious. For all the things I did for him, he didn't protect the little bit that I care about. But after he moved, I met him for lunch one day and he gave me a pair of toe shoes. All his therapy finally paid off. He was saying: "I know what's important to you. It *does* matter to me."

When Sara had to make a life and death decision about removing a ventilator from her father, it was harrowing but she never felt guilty about letting him die because she felt loving toward him. She had had the opportunity to tell him how she felt about him and he was able to respond in a way that made her feel heard.

They said he wouldn't last more than three minutes without a ventilator. I asked them to remove it. They pulled out the tube and he started gagging. It was horrible. I'm holding his hand. "Daddy I love you, Daddy I love you." It went on for *an hour.*

Eventually, after her father died, Sara's mother developed an infection and needed to be hospitalized. In the hospital, she forgot how to swallow and they asked to put in a feeding tube. Sara didn't know what to do. The doctor said: "Why don't you talk to some of your mother's old friends and see what they think?"

That was the best advice. They reminded me who my mother was and that she wouldn't have wanted this. I put her in hospice and the understanding was that there would be no feeding tube. She didn't eat for ten days and I felt that I was starving my mother to death.

Soon after her mother went to the hospice, Sara went to dinner with some colleagues and one woman said: "I would never put my mother in a nursing home." Sara felt guilty and horrible about her decision. But then there was another woman who helped Sara gain perspective.

I had a bad cold that day and she said: "You know how you're sick now and you're just pushing your food around on the plate, but you don't really want to eat? If I forced you to eat what's on your plate, that's what it's like putting a feeding tube in a person who's dying." It let me have a visceral idea of what it would mean to put the feeding tube in. The next day I got the phone call that she died. But the lingering feeling is: "Did I starve my mother to death?"

Sara feels guilty about her decision not to put in a feeding tube. Her anger makes her question her own motives. She asks herself, "Did I starve her to death because she starved me emotionally my whole life?" When you make life and death decisions for a parent, feeling angry increases the guilt if the choice is death. If you are feeling loving, as painful as it is to choose death, it is easier to feel that you are doing the right thing for your parent as well as yourself.

Sara explained that she wrote on her father's tombstone: "He got happy." Her father wasn't happy when he was young. But in the few years before he died, he found an assisted living facility and moved to the city. He went to the theater and made friends. These were things he never did before. Sara felt she had a part in her father being happier before he died because she was also able to work through some painful issues with him before he died. But she felt differently about her mother.

> With my mother [deep sigh], I haven't put anything on her gravestone yet because I can't think of anything positive to say. I went to her grave and asked her guidance for what I can say. But all I come up with is negative things. I have to lie, say nothing or say something very obtuse. There's no closure.

Her mother's Alzheimer's foreclosed the possibility of Sara working anything out with her mother before she died.

> When she first got Alzheimer's I went through a kind of mourning. I realized that I was never going to have the relationship with my mother that I always wanted. Once she had Alzheimer's I knew that was never going to happen. I wondered what I'd feel like when she died. To some degree it was a nonevent. There wasn't an "Oh, God she's dead."

Sara was left yearning for a relationship with her mother that she never had and never would have: "I see mothers and daughters on the subway chatting away and I know I will never have that."

Sara began to recall that her mother, who was a teacher, was always very depressed and that, as a child, she tried to take care of her mother.

I always felt I was the adult in the house. I'll take care of you, I'll entertain you; I'll make sure everything is okay. I remember sitting around the table—with my two aunts and feeling the tension. I felt that I had to make them get along. I had to make things right. I cooked dinner every night from the time I was eight or ten. I helped her grade. If something broke I fixed it. If we needed something, I'd run out and get it.

Sara understands that her mother's depression was rooted in a childhood experience. She explained that her mother was the apple of her grandfather's eye and then he lost his money in the Depression and was no longer functional. They had to move out of their house and relatives had to support them. Sara feels that experience of loss was a formative experience for her mother.

Sara went on to say that her mother was a businesswoman, but gave it up when she got married. She became a teacher so that she and her husband, who was a teacher, could have summers off together. But Sara explains that while her father loved teaching, her mother hated it. Her mother seems to have experienced giving up her career as another thing that she loved being taken away from her. She came home each day tired and angry; her mother acted out her feelings of resentment on Sara.

She had me grading her papers when I was a kid. My older sister was a rebel and she and my mother were always in battles, so I felt I had to be extra good to compensate for all the trouble my sister caused. Mom never said anything good to me. No matter what I did it was never good enough.

Sara tried to please her mother, but she never succeeded. Rather, her mother envied Sara because she loved dancing. Her mother couldn't stand Sara doing something she loved when she felt so deprived herself.

> I was a dancer as a kid. I was in a semiprofessional group. I loved it. She had this thing about me dancing. They wouldn't pay for dance class. I had to work in the dance studio to pay for my classes. She promised if I got good grades I could dance and then she didn't follow through. In the area that was my self, my center, she didn't support me—she got in the way.

Sara cried as she described her mother's broken promise. Her feelings of resentment toward her mother posed a particular problem when Sara had to make the decision about the feeding tube. The doctor said: "Just tell her you love her." But Sara couldn't do that; she felt too angry with her mother. She was angry for always having to be good to compensate for her sister being bad and not getting any appreciation for it anyway. She felt hurt and angry with her mother for not allowing her to dance. But the experience that seemed to hurt the most was her mother's response when her sister had a psychotic breakdown.

Sara had been very close to her older sister, Tammy. After the birth of her third child, at age thirty-one, Tammy had a postpartum depression. She called Sara and said her husband was tapping the phone and trying to kill her. Then her brother-in-law called Sara and told her all the insane things Tammy was saying. Sara flew to Chicago the next day and hospitalized her sister. Sara describes it as something she did entirely alone—without the help of her brother-in-law or either of her parents. Tammy didn't want to be hospitalized; she jumped out of the car and tried to run away. Sara says:

> It was the hardest thing I've ever done. When I came back, my mother said I hospitalized my sister because I was jealous. It was sibling rivalry. Later my sister had a second break and my mother finally went out there to visit her. Imagine, it took two psychotic breaks for my mother to go out there and see her. She still wouldn't believe her darling daughter was psychotic. It's very difficult to make care choices for someone you're angry with.

When her mother was in the nursing home, Sara's cousins told her she was giving her more love and caring than her mother ever gave her. Indeed, Sara had a second wedding ceremony at the nursing home so that her mother could be at her wedding. But she is still left with the nagging question: "Did I put her in the nursing home because it was the best thing or because I was angry? Did I decide to not give her the feeding tube because I wanted to kill her?" Making that decision for a parent is painful and difficult no matter how much you love them, but if Sara had a well of love to draw on, she might feel more confident about the answer. She might feel sad and pained rather than guilty.

Sara told me that she's had a recurrent dream for many years—she dreams that she is buried alive and people are walking around above not knowing she's there. That is how Sara felt about her parents—each one was walking around without knowing she was there. Neither of her parents was able to see Sara's needs—her need to be a child and not take care of her parents, her need to be told the truth and her need to dance. Her mother was sadistic toward her and her father did not protect her. Sara's anger toward her mother never got resolved, leaving Sara with guilt about putting her in a nursing home and not putting in a feeding tube. Her anger toward her father, on the other hand, was resolved, so the decision to remove the ventilator was difficult, but did not leave her with guilt.

THE GUILT THAT GOES WITH BEING THE SPECIAL ONE WHO IS FAR AWAY

"My guilt is that my mother is dying alone . . ." Tom is a fifty-three-year-old editor who lives in New York. About six months ago, his eighty-one-year-old mother, who lives in Denver, had a stroke and went to the hospital and then to a nursing home. She lost her speech as a result of the stroke and then developed pneumonia in the nursing home and is now back in the hospital suffering from kidney failure. When I interviewed Tom, he and his family were making a decision about whether to put his mother on dialysis or let her die.

Tom has three younger sisters, and it is his middle sister who is the primary caregiver. She lives close to their parents and is currently unemployed. She was with her parents when her mother had a stroke. She visits her several times a day and picks up her father every day, takes him to the hospital and drives him back home.

Tom feels that his mother is dying "alone" because he feels that he is the only person who understands her and the only one who can comfort her. He says:

You can see she's trying to smile, she tries to formulate a question, but it comes out as a grunt. In the four days I was there, she got better. When I arrived, she rolled over and said clearly: "I love you." My mother and I never had much of a physical relationship, but when I visited her I told her stories, rubbed her neck and her arms. My sister put cream on her arms, but this was different.

Tom explained that his father has never offered any comfort to his mother. He was physically and emotionally abusive to his wife and his children. Tom's mother was pregnant with him when she married his father and Tom does not think they would have gotten married otherwise. He describes his father as a "falling-down drunk." Although he told me that his mother did not intervene to stop his father's drinking or allow anyone else to, Tom identifies with his mother as a victim of his father. Tom says his mother never expressed her needs and his father viewed her entirely as existing to fulfill his. When she started to show symptoms of Alzheimer's, Tom's father wouldn't believe she didn't know something or couldn't remember it.

While Tom views his father as ignoring his mother's needs, he views himself as the person who always understood her. It is ironic that she lost her ability to talk because, as Tom says:

Even when she could talk, she never expressed her emotions. I only saw my mother cry once or twice in my whole life.

Nevertheless, Tom always felt that he intuitively understood his mother.

Once my mom was in the hospital, knowing my mother the way I do, she was probably very frightened about what was happening to her. Part of her mind was active and alive. I could see it when I visited her.

Tom's father says he can't stand seeing his wife unable to speak or understand anything so he doesn't like to visit her. He goes every day, but Tom feels angry toward him because he stays very briefly and clearly doesn't *want* to be there. Tom says:

He's so self-involved he can't imagine that she has a need to see him. The last day I was there I tried to explain this to him. I told him: "When you're there, she's responsive." But he's so self-involved, he says: "Nobody understands how hard this is. My body can't take it." He *never* in his life thought about anyone having needs except him.

Tom feels guilty that he is not with his mother because he feels that he could comfort his mother in a way that his father refuses to do.

I said: "Why can't you just sit in the hospital room and watch television together?" He says: "You don't understand how hard this is for me."

His guilt is intensified by his knowing the eldest of his sisters doesn't visit his mother and he feels that the middle sister, who visits her mother several times a day, cannot offer her the kind of comfort that he can offer. He chuckles when he tells me that his sister's boyfriend is named Tom and when he goes to visit his mother she smiles and is very responsive to him. He fantasizes that she thinks it's her son Tom.

> I had to help the nurse turn my mother over. I found myself holding my mother, she looked up at me and I knew she was comfortable, she felt safe. It was such a familiar feeling to be with her like this. I felt it was a regression back to this early place where we were together. I felt that I understood my mother on a level that my father and sisters never did.

Feeling that he has a special bond with his mother makes Tom feel guilty because he feels that he is the only one capable of offering her any comfort.

> There's a part of me that wanted to be there when my mother died. I felt guilty coming back to New York. I can't afford to take off from work and stay with her. I don't know how long it will take. Is it just my *fantasy* that my mother is alive and well inside this shell? I can't imagine anything worse than to go through the process of dying totally alone.

Without him, he feels, his mother is totally alone.

IT WOULD BE wonderful if as adults we could appreciate our own compassion and attempt to do the right thing for our parents. But despite their heroic efforts to take care of their parents, Sharon, Sara and Tom are all plagued with often crippling guilt. Their deep, unresolved feelings about their mothers leave them unable to get over the guilt. Sara's guilt is the result of unresolved anger toward her mother, while Sharon and Tom's guilt is based on feeling they didn't do enough for the loved parent for whom they have felt responsible since childhood. Each of them struggles with different degrees of guilt, unable to forgive themselves. Sharon can't forgive herself for not saving her mother. She is stuck in the relentless self-punishment of "If only I . . ." Sharon won't be able to forgive herself until she is able to empathize with the little girl who felt that her mother's life was in her hands.

Sara, on the other hand, does not torture herself with the wish to undo the decisions she made. She accepts them. She feels she would make the same decisions again. But making those decisions while still angry has left her with anxiety about her sadistic wishes toward her mother. She's left asking herself: Did I act on them? Sara won't be able to forgive herself until she is able to separate her wishes and her actions toward her mother. She may have wished, at moments, to hurt her mother. But her actions toward her mother were not sadistic. She did what she could for her—more than many daughters. She made a decision about the feeding tube based on her mother's quality of life *as well as her own,* but the latter doesn't cancel out the former. Adult children often feel guilty for decisions that give consideration to their own life circumstances. But relationships involve weighing the needs of both people—we do that with our children and we have to do that with our parents.

Tom feels guilty for not comforting his mother in her dying hour in a way he feels only he had the power to do. Tom has always felt merged with his mother—as if they are one.

Tom will only be able to forgive himself when he accepts his mother's separateness. He was able to say goodbye to her. She knew he came to say goodbye. That's all we can do for another person—even our mother.

While we all deal with feelings of guilt about cruel things said or inconsiderate behavior, neurotic guilt is not based on actually hurting another person. Yet, neurotic guilt can be debilitating and, because aspects of it are often unconscious, it is very difficult to talk someone out of it. It's neurotic! Then what can we do to reduce crippling guilt? How can we make peace with ourselves? Taking care of our elderly parents exacerbates our neurotic guilt, but using this stage of life as an opportunity to reduce it enriches us and enhances the rest of our lives.

Often we vacillate between anger and guilt, so trying to work out angry feelings with a parent reduces guilt. Of course, the most ideal way of working out those angry feelings is *with* the parent before he or she dies. Sara was able to do that with her father. Unfortunately, that is often impossible either because the elderly parent is no longer lucid or because he or she is unable to take any responsibility for hurting you. Feeling angry toward a parent with Alzheimer's is particularly difficult because their inability to comprehend your anger increases the guilt. In that case you may need a therapist to help you work out the angry feelings.

Second, when we hear ourselves use a lot of "shoulds" that is a tip-off that we are trying to meet other people's expectations of what we should do. It might be helpful to ask yourself: What do I think is right? What do I need to do in order to make peace with myself? There is no one prescription for dealing with difficult life milestones with an elderly parent. You have to find your own level of tolerance and clarify your own values.

For the adult child who feels only he can take care of Mom because he is the special child, ameliorating guilt is particularly difficult. There is a conflict between the wish to feel special and the wish to not feel guilty. Unfortunately, they are linked—if you are the only one who is special enough to take care of Mom then you will feel guilty for allowing anyone else to care for her. Reducing guilt involves giving up feeling special and allowing or encouraging other family members to participate in caregiving.

Finally, for those who feel guilty because they always criticized other people for putting their parents in nursing homes and now want to do it themselves, let this be a lesson in humility and compassion. It's much easier to make judgments about people when you are not in the same position. People change and life situations change. Before you had children or worked full-time you might have felt you wanted your parents to live with you when they needed care. But now your situation may have changed; you may have changed. Forgive yourself.

Part II

RELATIONSHIPS THAT OFFER SUPPORT OR CREATE CONFLICT

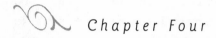 *Chapter Four*

SPOUSES

> My mother never liked my husband, and she was never
> nice to him, so he doesn't want to see her. I understand
> how he feels, but I am left with the burden by myself.
>
> —*A married caregiver*

AT SIXTY, my husband, Richard, still feels angry toward his
mother because she invited his grandmother to move in
when his grandfather died. The family of four lived in a
house with three bedrooms and Grandma was put in Richard's room—when he was five years old. Grandma stayed
there until he was ten. I was shocked that his parents put his
grandmother in their son's rather than their seven-year-old
daughter's room, but I am more surprised that Richard is
not angry at his father—only his mother. Richard says his father did not want his mother-in-law to live with his family,
but he never insisted that his wife and her brothers make
other arrangements for their mother. Instead, he permitted
Richard to share his room with his elderly grandmother.

Was Richard's father being a good husband or was he ab-
negating his responsibility as a husband and father? It's a

difficult question to answer—we have to examine our assumptions about what it means to be a "good husband" and "good father." There is not one universally agreed-upon answer to these questions—and our perspective changes over time. In the 1950s, when Richard was growing up in an upper-middle-class family, a good father and husband was one who was a good economic provider. Fathers were not expected to be involved in child care—men were supposed to go out to work, and women were supposed to stay home and take care of the children. Sixty-three percent of families in 1950 were composed of a wage-earning dad, a stay-at-home mom, and one or more children.[1] Richard's family fit the dominant demographic perfectly: his mother stayed home in the suburbs and his father took the Long Island Rail Road to work in New York City. Now only 17 percent of all American families conform to the tradition of wage-earning dad, stay-at-home mom and one or more children.[2]

Expectations of what it means to be a good husband and father have changed as more women entered the workforce. Since more than 70 percent of all married women with children under eighteen participate in paid labor outside the home, we have come to expect married men to do more than bring home a check.[3] As the economic structure changed so did the division of labor within the family. Husbands, especially upper-middle-class ones like Richard's father, are expected to share in the domestic chores and play a larger role in the care of their children. Fathers are expected to play an emotional role in the family, not simply an economic one. So what does this mean about Richard's father?

From the traditional 1950s point of view Richard's father *was* being a good husband and father, but his son was left feeling unprotected. From my point of view as a psycho-therapist, Richard's father failed him in a fundamental way. In a good marriage a spouse can help a caregiver realize that her mother is not her primary relationship anymore. The caregiver is no longer dependent on her mother as she was as a child. She has a husband to depend upon and a husband and children who depend upon her. Richard's father did not perform this important function as a husband/father. He complained about his mother-in-law, but he did not take action.

Husbands can also be helpful to a caregiver by helping her find a way to alleviate guilt. For example, Sara's husband was able to help her do what made her feel good about herself without losing herself.

I met my husband on a blind date and told him I had to leave to buy clothes for my mother, who was in a nursing home. He said: "Oh, can I come with you?"

Sara's husband was immediately comfortable with her role as caregiver. He joined her in it in a way that allowed her to marry him and still take care of her mother in a way that was part of her core identity.

When we got married, one of the decisions was whether we should get Mom from the nursing home and bring her to the wedding. I couldn't face putting her back in the nursing home after taking her out for a day. So my husband suggested: "Why don't we have a second wedding at the nursing home?" It ended up being wonderful for everyone. The day of the wedding there was a family support group meeting. People came up to me and said: "We haven't had any joy in this nursing home. Thank you for bringing some joy."

THE SPOUSE WHO ENABLES
THE LACK OF LIMITS

Remember Rose, from Chapter 1, who had such difficulty setting limits with her mother? Like Richard's father, Rose's husband, John, failed to help his wife set limits with her mother. Rose's husband did not even complain like Richard's father. Rose felt grateful that her husband did not pressure her to separate from her mother.

> My husband is a wonder. He has a lot of patience. I call him and say I don't feel like cooking, you better bring something in.

But Rose is unhappy having her mother live in her house. She feels controlled by her mother. She gave up her social life with her husband, daughters and friends for her mother: "She won't let us leave her alone, but when I tell her we're going out she doesn't want to go . . ." Rose's mother is using emotional blackmail on her. She is using her suffering as a way of making Rose feel guilty and manipulating her. As Susan Forward points out: "Becoming a caretaker to a sufferer is a full-time job."[4]

Rose feels she has no choice but to give in to her mother's demands; she feels victimized by her. Once, when she went out for dinner with her husband, her mother called 911, so they never did it again. Her mother's message is clear: "If you leave me I will suffer so much that you will be sorry." It would have been helpful to Rose if her husband, John, said,

"This is a problem, Rose. We can't live this way. The kids need to have a mother who can take them shopping or out to lunch. We need time alone together and I need to have a wife who isn't constantly drained and angry."

John has never done that. Rather, John seems to join Rose in her definition of the situation—that is, we have no choice but to do what Mother wants. John has never set any limits with his mother-in-law. She is living in his house, but he has never talked to her about the way she behaves. Rose says:

> He's not going to disagree with my mother. So she loves to see him. He goes in and she complains to him about me and he says: "I'll have to get after her about that." [She laughs.] He comes into the kitchen and laughs and tells me. I say to him, "You see what it's like to take care of her." [She laughs.] He's good. He's really good.

Rose's laughing does not feel like it's a response to something funny. When she says, "You see what it's like . . ." she shrugs, and I sense what she means is, "It's hopeless." She feels there's nothing that can be done to make the situation with her mother any better. But that's not true—that sense of hopelessness is a symptom of depression. John unknowingly adds to Rose's sense of hopelessness by going along with his mother-in-law's unreasonable demands rather than explaining to her that if she wants to live with his family, she has to make some compromises so that the situation will be more livable for them.

Rose does not understand John's role in her difficulties with her mother. She views his passivity as "helping." When he goes along with his mother-in-law's outrageous insistence that Rose and John cannot go anywhere without her, Rose experiences it as support rather than collusion: "He has no qualms about helping me pack her up to take her somewhere. He's real, real good. I manage."

Is Rose's husband a concerned partner or did he allow his wife to sacrifice important aspects of their marital relationship and their daughters' development? I think John *was* a concerned partner, but he seemed to make the same assumption as Rose—that they had no choice.

THE SPOUSE WHO HELPS SET LIMITS

Elizabeth and her husband, Tom, seem to have been able to set up a much more livable situation than Rose and John— although they gave up their home to move in with Elizabeth's mother. Elizabeth and Tom felt that they *had* options, but *chose* to live with Elizabeth's mother and take care of her. Elizabeth is a very striking woman with short white hair and a rather formal manner. She is fifty-seven years old and her husband, Tom, is sixty; they have two grown daughters. Born in a small town in Massachusetts, Elizabeth went to the University of Texas and then got a master's in counseling at the University of Pennsylvania.

I've been far from home since I was eighteen years old. That's the irony of it. I loved living in New York for all those years after school. My husband and I lived in a lovely neighborhood and knew everyone. I started a shelter for battered women and ran it for fifteen years.

Elizabeth talks with nostalgia about the years she lived in New York and ran a shelter for battered women. Her voice gets sad at the end when she adds: "Then my father died and my mother has very bad arthritis."

Elizabeth and her husband were running back and forth from New York to Amherst, Massachusetts, to check in on her mother. Then Tom got a job at a school in Massachusetts and Elizabeth kept her job in New York. Tom was living with her mother during the week; Elizabeth would join them on the weekend.

It's amazing, he never could have done that with my father or his own parents, but he always loved my mother and felt closer to her than to his own mother.

Tom's feelings for Elizabeth's mother were a key element in their caregiving. *He* wanted to care for her mother as much or more than Elizabeth did. In addition, Elizabeth did not like having a commuting marriage. She decided to give up her job and move to Amherst. She and Tom decided to buy her mother's house and live with her.

I asked Elizabeth what kinds of things she does for her mother.

I bathe her every night and my husband gives her breakfast and lunch because he's off for the summer. Then I make dinner for the three of us. She has good days and bad days—it's mostly related to the weather. On good days she can do a lot of things for herself, but on bad days she needs a lot of help. The problem is that you don't know when there will be a bad day. You can't plan in advance and you can't really be spontaneous either.

It sounds like a situation that could be quite dismal. But in contrast to Rose and John, Elizabeth and Tom manage to take care of themselves while taking care of her mother. Once a week a woman comes in and cleans the house and bathes her mother so that Elizabeth and Tom can go out.

And then every once in a while I call my sister and say: "I can't take it anymore, please come." She comes and we go away. Or my brother in New Hampshire will take her for two weeks and then we can go out to dinner and go bike riding and hiking while she's gone.

There are other ways in which Elizabeth and Tom have made the situation more livable. They have made the relationship more reciprocal by asking her mother for rent—that helps pay the mortgage and makes them feel that they are getting something back for taking care of her. In contrast to John, Tom supports Elizabeth by being clear with her mother about what they can tolerate when it is difficult for Elizabeth to do it.

She had cataracts and was losing her vision. The doctor said she needed an operation to have them removed, but she didn't want to do it. My husband and I felt that we could not live with her if she was blind—she'd have to go to a home. He told her that she had to have the operation.

She didn't want to and felt very resentful. But she had it and now she's fine.

Elizabeth talked about how painful it was to deal with her mother's resentment when she has made such a big sacrifice for her.

She complains to my sister and brothers about me. Of course, they understand the situation. Recently I increased my work hours to thirty-five hours a week. When I told her she said: "What's the difference? You never do anything for me anyway."

Although she didn't explicitly say it, I got the impression that Elizabeth was happy to work thirty-five hours a week. It's hard for her to be with her mother.

It's not easy. But sometimes I just say to my husband, I've had it. I'm going for a walk. You deal with her. And he does. It works because he does it with me; we do it together.

When Elizabeth says, "We do it together," she is not simply referring to the caregiving. What Elizabeth and Tom have been able to do is make the house *their* house—they bought the house rather than simply living in the house owned by her mother. As soon as they bought it, they ripped off the kitchen and built a new one. Elizabeth said that helped a great deal to allay the feeling that she was giving up her whole life and moving home with her mother.

But perhaps the most important element in allowing Elizabeth and Tom to take care of her mother and feel good about it is that Tom has helped Elizabeth set limits on her mother's control over their lives.

> She would tell me what to do in the garden or how to do it and I couldn't stand it. Finally, my husband said to her: "We can't live here if you tell us what to do. We're used to having our own house and our own garden." That really helped. She does it once in a while, but it's much better.

Elizabeth was getting angry at her mother's controlling behavior, but she could not talk to her about it. It was her husband who intervened on her behalf and made it possible for Elizabeth to tolerate living with her mother without being angry toward her all the time.

IN THE CASES I have described, the daughters were the caregivers and in both cases the husbands agreed to living with their mothers-in-law. Now let's turn to a situation in which the son is the caregiver and his wife resented his need to care for his mother.

THE ABANDONING SPOUSE

Tony counsels teenagers for a nonprofit community organization in Columbus, Ohio. The office is a tiny hole-in-the-wall with papers and books strewn everywhere. It's hard to find a place to sit. Tony is wearing a pair of wrinkled chinos and a short-sleeved shirt. He's a husky Italian-American man of forty-six. He is married with two children—a nineteen-year-old son and seventeen-year-old daughter.

Tony's mother has had lupus for over twenty years, but during the last five years of her life, it was debilitating and she was on oxygen and bedridden. Tony's stepfather was there, but Tony still felt that he had to be the primary caregiver for his mother.

It was really hard. I was working, trying to take care of my family and trying to be there for my mother. Especially because it was only a mile down the road, I passed her home every day and I felt I needed to be there. I tried to be there as much as possible—sometimes every other day. She lived with my stepfather, but we [he corrects himself], I took care of her.

Tony had a very special relationship with his mother because of his childhood. His parents divorced when he was a baby and his mother was left with two boys. When Tony was about eight years old, his mother couldn't deal with working full-time and caring for her two sons.

I lived away from my mother for about seven years from third grade to eighth grade—five years . . . I went with one grandmother and my brother went with the other grandmother. I didn't go visit my mother that often. You know, you get involved with your friends and stuff. Then I moved back with my mother and stepfather and we moved up here. It was hard that relationship at home—feeling like I should be in both places. It was difficult.

Tony tells me about his traumatic past very casually. He doesn't seem to think that being sent away by his mother, separated from his brother, taken out of one school and having to start at a new one, after he had already been abandoned by his father, had much of an effect on his life. Tony casts the story of being sent to live with his grandmother in an interesting way. He reverses the relationship between his mother (the adult at the time) and himself (the child at the time) when he says he didn't go to visit her very much because he was involved with his friends. He feels that even as a child it was his responsibility to take care of his mother; he is careful to hold his mother blameless for not visiting him! He seems to need to protect her.

Tony had a strong wish to be close to his mother once he was reunited with her as a result of her marrying his stepfather. When he married, Tony and his wife, Jan, bought a house down the road from his mother; he continued to feel a strong need to take care of her—perhaps as a result of his childhood experience as well as the tragic death of his older brother.

> He got shot fifteen years ago and ended up in a traumatic brain injury hospital. That was kind of difficult. So I was the only son left. He was hanging out in an after-hours bar with people that were known not to be reputable and had an argument with a guy over my brother's girlfriend and the guy pulled out a gun and shot him in the head. He died two years before my mother did.

Tony's wish to be close to his mother was intensified by his feeling that he had to be a "good kid" because his brother's brain injury, twelve-year hospitalization and subsequent death were so painful for his mother on top of her own illness.

He was not a good kid. He was a drug addict. When she was sick, I was the only one left. I was always the good kid. Even if I did something a little wrong, I didn't want to be like my brother.

There was always a split in the image of the two brothers—Tony, "the good kid," and Joey, "the bad kid." Tony lived with the expectation that he had to make up for his brother's badness with his goodness. Unfortunately, Tony's wife did not understand the psychological importance of Tony's taking care of his mother.

One of the other situations that really affected me was my wife and two kids just stepped back, away from the whole process. I felt like I was really alone. It's two years later and it's still there. It really changed our relationship—more with my wife than the kids.

Tony felt very conflicted about his obligation to his wife and children and his need to take care of his mother. He wanted Jan to understand how much he needed to care for his mother, but she didn't. Perhaps she felt abandoned by Tony because of the intensity of his involvement with his mother.

Jan wouldn't go visit at all. When my mother was in the hospital, I'd run down to visit her. She'd say: "Oh, you're going *again* . . ." Little things like that made me feel bad. I'd say, "Do you want to take a ride?" Even if she didn't want to sit in the room, she could have come for a ride with me. I'd only stay half an hour or so. My mother couldn't talk a lot, but she knew you were there and she appreciated you coming. That was really hard. When my mother passed away, I was there by myself.

I asked Tony if he and Jan had gotten any help to sort out what happened between the two of them when his mother was sick: "No, once in a while we talk about it, it's just there. We don't argue. We don't ever argue. It's just the way it is." I asked him why he doesn't seek help since he seems to be in chronic pain: "Yeah, I am. I don't know. With whatever goes bad, I just try to put it aside. I'm involved with kids."

I asked him if he thought there was any connection between feeling abandoned by his wife when his mother was sick and his experience of being sent to live with his grandmother as a child. I sensed Tony's depression and went further with him than perhaps I should have. I pointed out that the way he described doing other things to avoid the feelings of hurt and anger at his wife sounded similar to the way he described coping with his mother sending him to live with his grandmother.

> That's kind of deep. I think of it as just one of those things. That may be. I don't know. The way I deal with things is I don't give myself a lot of time to think about stuff—just keep moving. Overall, I'm a happy-go-lucky kind of person. I'm always smiling. Of course there's always that lingering pain there.

There was hopelessness in his laugh. He seemed to reject any possibility of other ways to understand his experience. He felt stuck. Tony did not seem very happy-go-lucky to me. On the contrary, he seemed like a hurt little boy who felt abandoned by his mother at eight and abandoned by his wife when he needed her most. But Tony seems to cope by giving others what he did not get from them.

> When my wife's parents were sick, I wanted to see her take care of them. I wanted to make sure that she went down and visited. I said to her: "You'll be sorry later if you don't do it." She wound up being there when her mother died last fall, because I pushed her to do that. I felt good about it. Now her dad is ill and she seems to have a different attitude. So hopefully, little by little we'll build that whole thing back up.

Tony's view of his problems with Jan is that she did not understand the importance of caring for elderly parents— his or her own and that made him feel abandoned by her when he was caring for his mother. Tony seems to believe that by Jan caring for her dad in a way Tony deemed appropriate, the trust in the marriage will be rebuilt. However, Tony never talked to Jan about how he felt about what he experienced as her lack of support during the last years of his mother's life. He still doesn't talk to Jan about how he feels about that experience and how it has changed their relationship. Jan has never talked to Tony about how she felt about him spending so much time away from her and their children in order to care for his mother. Perhaps she felt that he was overly involved with his mother's care. But Tony says she never discussed that with him, she just made hostile remarks like: "Oh, you're going *again*."

From my experience as a psychotherapist, it seems unlikely that trust can be rebuilt without talking about the breach and understanding what each of them was going through at the time. Very likely both Tony and Jan are hurting. Just as Tony may have experienced Jan's lack of support as a repetition of his childhood experience of being sent away by his mother, Jan may have experienced Tony's absences as a repetition of an early experience in her life. Intractable marital problems often involve unconscious repetitions of childhood traumas. Unearthing the meaning of the empathic failures and the depth of the pain is difficult without the help of a therapist.

THE IMPORTANCE OF THE SPOUSE WHEN THE CAREGIVER IS AN ONLY CHILD

Jonathan is a fifty-year-old only child. He is married to Barbara, who is an accountant. Jonathan recently went back to school to fulfill a lifelong dream of becoming a social worker. I interviewed him twice over a period of two years of caregiving and I interviewed Barbara as well. When I first interviewed Jonathan he was living two hours from his parents' house. His mother, Betsy, who has bipolar disorder, was eighty years old at the time. She had had a knee replacement and needed another. His father had coronary heart disease and advanced cancer of the bladder which metastasized to his liver. His father needed oxygen, but his cancer was in remission.

Jonathan felt angry because he and his wife, Barbara, had been trying for years to get his parents to move into an assisted living facility in Brooklyn. That would make it easier for Jonathan to visit them and it would make the adjustment easier for the survivor when one of them died. Jonathan's

Dad thought it was a good idea. But Jonathan says: "My mother's the one who dug in her heels and said: 'No, I'm not doing it.' So I was really mad at her."

When Jonathan's father was diagnosed with cancer, his parents needed extensive help in the home. Jonathan kept trying to get his mother to take some responsibility and make decisions, but his mother *could not* do it. Jonathan felt she *would not* do it. That made him angry at her. He ended up making many decisions about hiring help, but he felt angry at his mother for not cooperating. Jonathan set up homecare for his father. He had a bathroom put in on the ground floor and set up a downstairs bedroom area for his father. He hired someone to shop, clean and cook.

Jonathan's father died a year and a half ago. Only then did Jonathan and his wife, Barbara, realize how much his father had been taking care of his mother. Despite all of Jonathan's efforts to create support for his mother, she had a major depressive episode a few months after his father's death and she had to be hospitalized. Jonathan devoted himself entirely to getting appropriate treatment for his mother. She was first put into the psychiatric ward of a general hospital near her home in New Jersey. Jonathan was driving back and forth from Brooklyn to the hospital in New Jersey on an almost daily basis or sometimes staying over at his mother's house. But Jonathan felt that she was not getting the appropriate combination of therapy and medication there and was able to get her transferred to a hospital that specialized in geriatric psychiatric disorders.

When Betsy was ready to leave the hospital, Jonathan had to face the problem of where his mother would live. Barbara has been helpful to him by pointing out that his mother is not capable of making any decisions. She explains to him that his mother is not willfully *refusing* to make a decision; she is simply overwhelmed by the prospect. It was probably that fear of being overwhelmed that made her reject the idea of moving to an assisted living facility before her husband died.

It was clear to Jonathan and Barbara that Betsy was not able to live on her own. Jonathan's mother needed help to ensure that she took her twice-daily medications; she needed meals provided and transportation to her doctors' appointments. Therefore, when his mother was getting shock treatments, while Jonathan was visiting her and dealing with the doctors, Barbara was looking at two possible assisted living facilities that are located near their house. Once the decision between the two facilities was made, Barbara made the arrangements for her mother-in-law to move.

Jonathan makes all the medical appointments, medical decisions, etc.

> Barbara has been phenomenal. We complement each other. I'm not interested in the financial aspects and she's not interested in the medical, psychological, social aspects. It's burdensome for Barbara, but she's not being asked to step out of her comfort zone in terms of her skills and her emotional makeup. We've worked well as a team.

Jonathan and Barbara's caregiving roles are an example of gender role reversal. Jonathan does the emotional nurturing, while Barbara takes care of the practical tasks like paying bills, estate management, etc.

Aside from her ongoing psychiatric problems and increasing dementia, Jonathan's mother eventually had a second knee replacement. So there have been many medical appointments and decisions. His mother doesn't understand what the doctor tells her, so Jonathan has to speak to the doctor. Barbara says Betsy is someone who can carry on a wonderful conversation and be quite charming. She *appears* to understand what the doctor is telling her, but she doesn't really process it. It is not clear whether her lack of comprehension is the result of intense anxiety or dementia, or some combination of the two. But Barbara says: "What that means is that even if she tries to convey what the doctor says to us it doesn't make any sense."

Barbara says that Jonathan can immediately tell when his mother isn't listening or doesn't know what is going on. He gets angry at her, trying to get her to focus on a problem or make a decision. Jonathan says that led to a confrontation in a restaurant. He kept asking his mother to answer his question about what she wanted and his mother finally said, "You're badgering me. Stop badgering me." Jonathan says:

> My mother took a lot of lumps in the beginning. We had one pretty heated scene in a restaurant one night where she was crying and I was crying. [Bursts out laughing.] One of the people in the next booth had an expression on her face as if she were wondering: "What are these crazy people doing?"

Jonathan knows that is not the right way to talk to his eighty-two-year-old mother. He chides himself for losing his temper, but also feels justified. "From a therapeutic standpoint it sucked. It was a dumb thing to do. But I had to get those things out."

Barbara offers Jonathan support by listening to him ventilate. But she also steps in to mediate between Jonathan and his mother. She says that Jonathan's mother's approach to life is to want problems to go away rather than confronting them. She does not want to make decisions.

> She will say "yes" to everybody without actually dealing with the issue at hand. When Jonathan hears that, he knows she is not paying attention or understanding what's happening, and it throws him into a tizzy. He will say: "Mom, you really *have* to understand."

Barbara explains to Jonathan that, at this point, his mother does not *have* to understand. He has to make the decision without her understanding.

> Jonathan tries to make her understand some fairly complicated things and then she gets more and more frustrated and breaks down in tears.

What makes it so hard for Jonathan to accept that his mother is not capable of understanding certain issues or making decisions for herself? He wants to feel his mother *could* be more independent because otherwise he has to face her total dependence on him. He has been worrying about his mother since he was a little boy. As a child, Jonathan had to deal with a mentally ill mother.

> I was ashamed to have my friends come to the house because my mom was in a bathrobe and a shower cap and all

the curtains were drawn in the house. She would get so depressed, that she could barely move. She'd get my father off to work and make us breakfast. Then she'd go upstairs, lock the door, draw the shades, lie on the floor, and she kept a bottle of whiskey under the desk. And when she'd wake up, she'd take a drink of alcohol. Just enough to get her into a semicomatose state and she would just lie on the floor.

Jonathan's mother was misdiagnosed as a schizophrenic and went through extensive hospitalizations. She was away for months at a time when he was a child. She tried to kill herself more than once. Jonathan says:

I saw the scars on her wrists. Fortunately, it was a cry for help. Meaning she didn't go real deep. They were fairly superficial cuts. She tried to drink lye. She *did* drink lye. Then she tried to do herself in with pills. She underwent extensive convulsive therapy; she was medicated improperly. It wasn't until the mid-seventies that she found a psychiatrist who understood bipolar disorder and prescribed lithium.

When Jonathan was nineteen, his mother tried to kill herself with an overdose of pills. He says:

I could tell when she was going into a depressive cycle. I could look at her and I could see it coming and I could predict it. One day I was looking for my mother and I knocked on the door, and I heard a little voice. The door was locked. I said: "Open the door!" And then I realized there was an empty pill bottle on the floor.

Jonathan has good reason to wish that his mother could take care of herself and let him focus on his own life. However, it has kept him constantly angry at his mother. Barbara mediates and sometimes intervenes to stop the escalation. She says:

My mother-in-law, and my father-in-law when he was alive, have always seen me as more like them than Jonathan. They have always seen me as someone who was more on their wavelength than he is.

Barbara tries to use Betsy's sense of camaraderie with her to be a calming influence. She lets her vent her frustration with Jonathan as well as trying to get Jonathan to give up his fantasy that his mother can live independently.

Barbara's support role is particularly important for Jonathan because he is an only child. She says:

There is no one else to help him out other than me. So I am a second caregiver. I pay all of Betsy's bills. I arranged the move from her house in New Jersey to the assisted living facility. I unpacked all of the cartons and set up the apartment for her and I take care of all the financial and administrative issues.

The facility is close to Barbara's office so she picks up Betsy's mail while she is at a rehabilitation hospital recuperating from knee surgery, and if there is a problem with anything at the assisted living facility, they call Barbara.

Barbara seems to be setting more limits on her participation in the caregiving process. For example, Betsy went into the rehabilitation hospital last Wednesday and Barbara has been there once, while Jonathan has been there four times. She says:

> One of the hardest things as a spouse is that you are being relied on in many ways, but you don't have any decision-making power. When it comes right down to it, I'm not the child. It's *his* mother. He has the final say.

She says that Jonathan is only now beginning to see that his mother "doesn't get it" and can't make decisions. Earlier Jonathan wanted to help his mother to become an independent woman and he got angry at her when she did not.

> He wanted to give her the opportunity to make a decision, but she goes into a panic if she has to make a decision. For example, while decorating her apartment, she had a manic episode because she had to make decisions about colors and fabrics. She called the decorator at 5:45 a.m. on a Friday to ask her if she were coming to her house in a little while. When the decorator told her she wasn't coming that day but on Monday, she got very argumentative with her.

Jonathan has been working on accepting that his mother cannot be more independent.

> I've come to realize that, although I want her to be more self-sufficient, it's not going to happen. It never was and is not going to be. I seem to be learning and relearning that lesson.

He is learning to accept who his mother is, and in many ways always has been, and to be more accepting of himself as well. When he says he's "learning and relearning that lesson," he seems to forgive himself for not responding perfectly to his mother every time. But he is proud of his progress.

> One of her friends called and said: "Your mother's coming home tomorrow and the refrigerator is empty. What should I buy?" I called my mom and told her about it. She said: "That's a good idea." But I could hear the hesitancy in her voice. I said: "Well, what should I tell her to buy?" I knew my mother was having an anxiety attack over this decision. I didn't get angry at her.

Another problem is that it is hard for Jonathan to distinguish between cries for help to which he needs to respond immediately and whimpers that do not require him to rush to his mother's house. Jonathan has had years of practice being attuned to nuances of his mother's voice. Barbara says Betsy often calls to complain to Jonathan and he feels he has to immediately drop everything and visit her. Barbara reminds him that his mother may *want* him to visit, but that is not the same as *needing* him to take care of something. Before his father died, Jonathan promised to care for his mother. So he has to struggle with his guilt and sense of obligation as well as his anxiety that his mother is capable of regressing very quickly. Barbara says that Jonathan is in a perpetual state of expecting the worst. Every time the phone rings and it's *not* his mother or *about* his mother, he takes a sigh of relief. Nevertheless, Barbara says Jonathan is getting more able to say no to his mother without getting angry at her.

With Barbara's help, Jonathan is accepting his mother's limitations. Accepting that his mother cannot take care of herself and cannot make decisions for herself has helped Jonathan forgive her for the pain she put him through when he was a child. He is coming to realize that she really didn't have any control over her behavior. She failed him, but not because she wasn't trying or didn't love him.

WE HAVE SEEN the important role the spouse can play, but often doesn't, in helping the caregiver negotiate the relationship with the elderly parent. Richard's father and Rose's husband stood by as their wives' inability to set limits intruded on their family's happiness. On the other hand, Elizabeth's husband, Tom, was extremely helpful to her because he was an equal partner in caring for her mother and helped Elizabeth set limits with her.

Tony and Jonathan are atypical caregivers because they are sons caring for their mothers. Tony's story illustrates the negative impact that caregiving can have on a marriage if the spouses do not have the same expectations about caring for their parents and do not negotiate their differences. In contrast to Tony, Jonathan's wife was willing to share the burden of caregiving. She never took it over, he remains the primary caregiver, but she offered support to Jonathan and was sympathetic to his being an only child.

Chapter Five

SIBLINGS

"Hi Mom."

"Hi."

"Did you get the flowers for Mother's Day?"

"Yes, and Phil is so wonderful. He's so nice to everyone, and everyone talks about him. He's just so good to me."

I can feel my blood pressure going up. I feel the rage rising in my chest. I get off the phone quickly. I'm trying not to cry.

"I'll see you tomorrow, Mom."

"Oh good, great, I'll see you then."

The tears well up. I'm fifty-nine years old and I still feel unappreciated by my mother.

TAKING CARE OF YOUR PARENTS may strengthen the bonds with your siblings and intensify your sense that you can count on them. Our relationships with siblings are our longest, offering many opportunities to understand and work out unresolved issues that remain from childhood. This becomes critical in times of crisis, such as a parent's sudden illness or gradual decline. A group of siblings can become a team offering one another support and helping set limits. If there are only two siblings, they can be partners and divide the emotional and/or financial burden.

However, as Stephen P. Bank and Michael D. Kahn point out in *The Sibling Bond,* the early sibling relationship gets reactivated as elderly parents require extensive care.[1] In her book *Brothers and Sisters: How They Shape Our Lives,* Jane Mersky Leder describes the way that childhood relationships exert power over our adult sibling relationships.

> The quickness with which all the "stuff" from childhood can reduce adult siblings to kids again underscores the strong and complex connections between brothers and sisters. We can enter a family gathering as confident adults and exit feeling as unsettled as we did during childhood. Our siblings push buttons that cast us in roles we felt sure we had let go of long ago—the baby, the peacekeeper, the caretaker, the avoider.[2]

The most frequent conflicted sibling relationship that gets reawakened when elderly parents need help is sibling rivalry, and the most common brother-sister conflict relates to the splitting of responsibility and authority. The sister is the one most likely to have the day-to-day responsibility, while the brother is most likely to be seen as the authority (that is, the one who has the power of attorney, is executor of the will and makes the major financial decisions). In most families there is one primary caregiver who is responsible for the care of the parent. The vast majority of them receive little or no help from their siblings. For a female, having all male siblings greatly decreases the chances of getting help.[3] Thus, when siblings are of different genders, there is an interplay of gender roles and psychodynamics.

You may assume that daughters were more likely to care for their parents "in the old days" when fewer women were employed outside the home. But research has shown that college-educated women who have worked continuously throughout their adulthood are more likely than homemakers to become caregivers.[4] Just as most women add on a second shift when they work outside the home, retaining their role as primary parent and continuing to do the majority of the housework, female caregivers who work outside the home add on a third shift. While being employed reduces the average level of a son's caregiving by twenty hours a month, having a job does not reduce the level of his sister's assistance.[5]

Discussions comparing the way sisters and brothers care for elderly parents parallel discussions of the gendered division of labor between husbands and wives. Husbands are more likely to undertake tasks that have clear and identifiable boundaries (for example, mowing the lawn) and tasks that have greater discretion in how and when to complete them (for example, minor household repairs). Wives, on the other hand, are more likely to take responsibility for aspects of family life that do not have clear and identifiable boundaries—keeping up relationships with family and friends, making sure the children are happy in school, etc. They also take primary responsibility for tasks that must be performed on a regular basis such as shopping, cleaning, bathing the children and cooking. Brothers and sisters divide caregiving responsibilities along similar lines.[6]

In her book *Respecting Your Limits While Caring for Elderly Parents,* Vivian Greenberg points out:

Over the years I have been struck by how much more difficult it is for daughters than for sons to set limits. As a result, caregiving is a more stressful experience for them
than for their male counterparts. In an effort to be "good
daughters" they place their needs secondary to those of
their parents.[7]

Compared to sons, daughters use less replacement support and are more involved in their caregiving role.[8] Hence,
sisters are more likely than brothers to experience caregiving
as stressful. And the stress of the caregiver role tends to
spill over to other aspects of the caregiver's life—for example, employment and family.[9] When compared to noncare-
givers, female caregivers average three times as many stress
symptoms, take more tranquilizers and antidepressants, and
report substantially less participation in social and recre-
ational activities.[10] Most important, daughters remain preoccupied with their parent's well-being even when not actually
rendering instrumental assistance. In the daughter's eyes, caregiving (like mothering) is a boundless, all-encompassing activity rather than a clearly demarcated set of discrete tasks.
For caregiver daughters, the dominant element (and burden)
in their caregiving is not the particular chores they perform,
but the continual sense of responsibility for their parents'
emotional state. Women are simply more likely to *notice* a parent's emotional state. Sisters are much more likely than their
brothers to be attuned to feelings and provide the emotional
work of caring for elderly parents.[11]

When there are brothers and sisters, one of the sisters
usually becomes the primary caregiver. Which sister becomes
the primary caregiver is sometimes the result of geographic

proximity. Frequently, adult offspring live far away from their parents. Only one-third of children aged forty-five to fifty-four live within fifty miles of their mothers (who might be married, divorced or widowed).[12] They may have moved away from where they grew up or their parents may have moved to another state in search of sun and leisure activities.

This makes it difficult for middle-aged children to manage their parents' care when they develop a chronic illness or become disabled. The burden usually falls on the sister living closest to the parents. Fifty percent of older parents live within five miles of their closest child—and the closest child is usually a daughter.[13] In these situations, the brother, often physically distant, tends to be given the authority in the parent's life, while his sister does the day-in and day-out caring for her parents.[14] The sister is left feeling unappreciated by her mother and angry toward her brother, who does little, but is idealized by their mother. For example, Gertrude is a seventy-two-year-old English teacher in a private school in Columbus, Ohio. She has a Ph.D. in English education and was chairperson of the English Department for many years. The day I interviewed her, her large dining room table was piled with term papers waiting to be graded. She describes her one-hundred-year-old mother's condition:

> My mother is physically very well, but she can't remember who I am. Sometimes she thinks I'm her sister—she asks me about Momma and Papa.

Gertrude's brother is five and a half years younger. The age and gender difference created a great deal of distance between them. Nevertheless, there is still competition. Gertrude told me that her brother is "a well-known professor" and when he is in town he visits his mother once a week and has lunch with her. However, he is rarely in town because he is often on leave, going to conferences and giving lectures. She feels that he assumes that his work is more important than hers.

Gertrude carries the emotional burden of caring for her mother.

> I pay the bills; go to the butcher; buy her underwear; pay the women who care for her. I call her every day. I would say he's involved minimally. He just went on an eight-month sabbatical. *They were away for eight months!* He came back three days after her stroke. I wrote him a note thanking him for the gift they brought me from their trip and telling him that I'm going to my college reunion next weekend. I got a message on my answering machine saying that he was going to Cleveland for the weekend. So he basically assumes I'm taking care of things.

When I asked Gertrude how it feels to be the one who takes care of things, at first she said what she feels is expected: "I don't mind doing it . . ." But then she added her feelings of resentment:

> I don't like the fact that he feels he can go and do whatever he wants and never tell me or ask me if it interferes with my plans. I don't think that if he knew what I was going to do that he would consider it when making his own plans. I happen to be a very loyal and conscientious person. I do what has to be done. Somebody has to do it.

Thus, it seems that overall the traditional expectations ascribed to male and female children are still intact for Gertrude and her brother. The experience of caring for her elderly mother has revived Gertrude's childhood feelings about differential expectations and treatment of her and her younger brother when they were children.

Gertrude and her brother are acting out their traditional roles in a family script in which every member has an internalized set of expectations. The current relationship is filtered through the internal one from the past. This is not limited to different gender-related expectations. For example, my friend Esther explained to me that her younger sister had always been sickly and her parents viewed everything she did in the context of overcoming adversity. Esther, on the other hand, was viewed as someone who had things easy and didn't exert herself. For Esther, these mental representations of herself and her sister continue into the stage of caregiving. Her sister views her professional work and family obligations as so taxing that finding time to care for her mother with Alzheimer's is almost impossible. On the other hand, she views Esther's professional work and family obligations as more flexible and less time consuming. Esther accepts this definition of herself, although it makes her angry. It feels "natural" to her. As a result, Esther spends much more time caring for her mother than her sister does and continues to feel a festering resentment at the inequity with which the burden is shared.

Esther and her sister illustrate that sibling relationships are not simply between the siblings, but they can also never be separate from the relationship to the parents. Sibling relationships take place in the context of a "family script" that involves a complex set of relationships between each child and each parent and each child in relation to the other children and each parent. We can see this more clearly when we look at the relationship between Karen and Robert.

CREATING A SIBLING CONNECTION THROUGH CAREGIVING: CHANGING OLD PATTERNS

Karen, Robert and Jane all live in the same small town where their mother lives, but until their mother got sick, they had very little to do with one another. I interviewed Karen and Robert. The social worker at the senior center suggested that I talk to them, but discouraged me when I suggested that I also call Jane; Robert and Karen similarly discouraged me from calling their sister. As a result, I can only include whatever I was able to glean about Jane's role in the family based on my interviews with Karen and Robert.

Karen is a forty-one-year-old married woman with two children. Although her older sister and brother are college graduates, Karen got married after high school and works part-time cleaning houses. She is a warm, pleasant woman who lives in a neat suburban house that is part of a subdivision.

Karen's mother had to organize her family's life around her husband's illness: Karen's father was diagnosed with cancer when she was a year old and he died when she was twelve.

Karen's mother cared for him all those years. Now, at seventy-three, her mother is dying.

> The last six months have been very bad . . . She couldn't get out of bed, couldn't eat, messes in the bathroom that I had to clean up. She's in the hospital now. She has pneumonia.

Karen feels that she has to take care of her mother the way her mother took care of her father.

> I still feel like I'm supposed to take care of my mother. I have this whole thing in my head. She took care of my father. She took care of my grandmother.

Karen strongly identifies with her mother as a caregiver to her father and grandmother, and because Karen's father was diagnosed with cancer when she was one, Karen's needs got lost somewhere. Her mother must have been distraught; she had already experienced two major losses and a trauma.

> My mom lost two babies, a boy and a girl. She gave birth and they died. One lived three hours and one lived three days. When my sister came along she had a cleft palate, so she needed extra care.

When Karen was born, Jane was two years old and Robert was eight years old. In between, their mother had two stillbirths and then gave birth to a baby with a cleft palate, Jane. Very likely she was depressed and overwrought by the series of traumas. Then within a year of Karen's birth, her father was diagnosed with cancer. There was not much of a chance for Karen to get her mother's focused attention. But what made it even worse was that the other two siblings did not nurture Karen either. They did not become a support system for one another as a result of their father's illness and mother's distraction. Rather, they remained emotionally isolated from each other, each one trying to get whatever they could from their parents and discounting one another.

> Recently, I'm finding out that Jane was Daddy's little girl. She's always hated my father, but now I realize she hated him for leaving. I was talking with my uncle about it . . . Robert was the apple of my mom's eye and Jane was the apple of my dad's eye.

If her sister was the apple of her father's eye and her brother was the apple of her mother's eye, and her mother was taken up with caring for her father, what happened to Karen? She was depressed. She describes symptoms of her childhood depression to me, although she doesn't name it as such.

> My sister says my mom yelled all the time when she was a child. I don't remember that. I slept all the time when I was a child. I don't know why.

Although she describes it to me, Karen does not seem to be in touch with how alone she felt as a child:

> When my mom knew that my dad was about to die, she sent my sister and I to my uncle's in Virginia for a couple of weeks. I remember my aunt coming into the little room where we were watching television and she said: "Your father passed away." I just went to my room and started crying. That was it really. I don't know how my sister and

brother reacted. My brother was twenty—he was in school.

Karen does not think it's strange that her mother sent her daughters away just before their father was about to die. None of the children were with him when he died. Karen was with her sister when she learned that her father died— but she went to her room in her uncle's house and cried alone. Her mother was not there to hug her and she could not emotionally connect with her sister, even at that moment. It made me teary to hear the story, but Karen told it matter-of-factly.

In *The Sibling Bond,* Stephen P. Bank and Michael D. Kahn point out that "sibling access" is a major determinant of the emotional bond between brothers and sisters. When siblings appear to have little emotional impact on one another, it's called "low access." Differences in age and sex diminish access by lessening the likelihood of common life experiences. Low-access siblings are often separated by more than eight or ten years, acting almost like members of different generations. In the case of Karen and Robert, they were six years apart. They had shared little time, space or personal history; they went to different schools and had different friends. They lacked a sense of shared history.

In addition, their parents discouraged them from creating an emotional bond and needing one another.[15] Sending Karen and Jane away and encouraging Robert to stay at college when their father was dying was a way of emotionally isolating the members of the family from one another. This kind of emotional isolation must have been typical for the family because Karen and Jane were only two years apart and they were physically together when they got the news of their father's death, but Karen went off and cried by herself and said she had no idea how Jane reacted. They did not feel that they needed each other.

In her loneliness, Karen turned to cleaning. Cleaning was a way of taking care of her mother and a way of feeling needed by her.

> My mother babied my sister and did everything for my sister. My sister never cleaned. She says she doesn't know how to clean. I always enjoyed cleaning. I would clean for my mother.

Karen defended against her aching by taking care of her mother and later in life it extended to other people. In fact, she told me that when her mother dies she is going to volunteer to clean the houses of old people. She said it made her feel good. Instead of experiencing her own wish to be taken care of, she helps others. And through her kindness, she can identify with the people she cares for so well.

Karen resisted setting limits on her caregiving even when it impinged upon her own children.

> I have an eight-year-old and a twelve-year-old. I could leave them home a little bit. But if I went to my mom's for fifteen minutes, it could be three hours later that I got home. I was over there all the time. When the kids were in school, I would drop them at school and go over there. I found this summer . . . was very hard—a real struggle. The guilt

of not being with my mom and having my kids . . . I was juggling all that.

The social worker at the senior center told Karen that she needed to take care of her husband and children.

Mom took care of my dad until the day he died. I said that to Bonnie [the social worker at the senior center] and she said: "Yes, that was her husband. But this is your husband. This is your mom but you have a family of your own."

Karen felt that Bonnie "gave her permission" to take care of her own family without feeling guilty about her mother. Bonnie represented the "good mother" who helped Karen set limits. Having a husband and two children was not enough for Karen to give herself permission to set limits caring for her mother. The event that enabled Karen to seek help from Bonnie was her husband's sickness. She became overwhelmed as a caregiver to both her mother and her husband. With Bonnie's help, Karen was able to transfer her identification with her mother as caregiver to her father, to her mother as caregiver to her own husband.

My husband just went through angioplasty. I took him to the emergency room at three o'clock in the morning. He woke me up and said: "I don't know, but I think I want to go to the hospital. I'm having these pains in my chest."

At that point in our conversation, Karen's eight-year-old son, Johnny, who had been listening intently for the last few minutes, corrected her.

No, Mom you took him to the hospital at three o'clock in the morning the first time, and then the second time, when he needed the angioplasty, it was just before I had to go to school.

Reflecting his anxiety about his father's health, Johnny knew every detail of his father's medical problems. Karen accepted his amendment to the story and continued:

The family doctor said to him that he couldn't keep putting off these tests. She scared him enough to take the test—an angiogram. When it was over the doctor came out and said we had two options—bypass surgery or angioplasty. He recommended angioplasty. I realized then that I'm needed here. I realized if my mom needs more care, we'll get it for her.

Despite her own childhood experience with a sick father, Karen did not seem to realize that her children would be deeply affected by their father's illness and Karen's over-involvement with her mother. Karen was unable to separate from her mother. She said: "I realized then that I'm needed here." She never realized that before because her mother was the center of her universe. Karen's desperate need to take care of her mother is rooted in her wish to be special to her mother in a way that she never was as a child. As a result, her son has his own separation problems. Johnny has developed a phobia about leaving the house because he has an insecure attachment to his mother as a result of her inability to separate from her mother. She whispered, so that her son could not overhear:

It helped me set my priorities. My son is having a very bad problem with everything going on. I explained to the pediatrician and she said she wants me to take him to a psychiatrist . . . He doesn't want to go to anyone's house. It's happened since Grandma went downhill and my husband has been sick.

Karen has been able to set limits on her mother's care, but only because she has transferred her need to be needed to her husband and her son. Unfortunately, instead of fostering a healthy sense of self and the confidence to move out into the world, the message to Karen's son is that the only way he can engage his mother is to stay home and need her to take care of him.

Karen's twelve-year-old daughter, Sarah, on the other hand, has developed a way of coping with her mother's absence that is based on her identification with her mother— she has become a caregiver. Her best friend has juvenile diabetes and she goes to the doctor with her and cares for her. When her friend went to an out-of-town hospital for medical tests she joined her for the trip. Unfortunately, Sarah and Johnny do not seem to have developed a supportive sibling bond. Sarah seems to spend most of her time away from home caring for her friend, while Johnny remains home suffering from intense anxiety.

One major reason for Karen's reluctance to turn to her brother for help is her internalized representation of Robert as distant and uninterested in her. Her complementary self-representation is as a needy child with nothing to offer her big brother. He is older, but he never took care of her. He stayed away from home as much as possible. Since he was the only boy and his mother's favorite child, Karen felt she could not compete with Robert; she could only clean in the hopes of getting her mother to love her. She has always seen Robert as powerful, distant and rejecting.

As a result of the consultation with Bonnie, Karen turned, for the first time, to her brother, Robert, for help. Robert is a forty-nine-year-old single man. He's tall and heavyset and seems uncomfortable and on edge. As I sat at the conference table in his office, I wondered why he volunteered to be interviewed. He seemed reluctant to talk, almost angry. He told me that he, Karen and Jane were never very close; he said they have nothing in common.

Although the three siblings were brought up in the same family and live within a mile of one another, Robert feels that they are all totally different—he "disidentifies" with both his sisters. In *The Sibling Bond,* Bank and Kahn point out that the disowning is usually the prerogative of the most favored child. It is unilateral—the privilege of the entitled child. Robert was the eldest child, the only son and his mother's favorite. He had the longest time with his father before he became ill. He monopolized the family's meager emotional riches and refused to protect his younger sisters. Instead, he felt superior to them and avoided uniting with them. He chose to stay at college when his father was about to die.[16]

Robert's interest in theater, which developed during the years of his father's illness, was another way of setting himself off from his sisters, and a way of distracting himself from what was going on at home. He went to school and stayed there for rehearsals after school, evenings and weekends. The "theater family" replaced his own family. Immersing himself in fantasy with a group of supportive teachers and friends must have been a welcome escape from his father's dying and his mother's depression. Although he did not make theater his career, he is still very active as an amateur. For Robert, the theater "is his life." He is not married, and until his mother got sick, he did not view his sisters as part of his life. At the end of the interview Robert said that he and Karen do love each other and they both love their mother and are trying to get the best care for her. Caring for their mother has given Robert more empathy for Karen.

I interviewed Robert when his mother was in the hospital—about two weeks before she entered a nursing home. He described his mother's condition:

> She went into the hospital because she had pneumonia, and broke her leg while she was there. She can't be left alone, and despite all of Karen's efforts and visiting nurses for the past year, there are periods when she's alone and in danger. She doesn't take her medicine properly, she loses her balance and falls, and her personal hygiene is getting worse.

Robert told me that his mother was going downhill and he convinced his sisters, despite Karen's reluctance, that she had to go into a nursing home when she got out of the hospital. He does not want Karen to be left with the burden of his mother any longer. He is worried about her, but knows that Jane will not offer her help and he feels that he cannot give the time that it would take to help Karen care for her if their mother went back home.

Jane lives in her mother's house. As Robert puts it: "She just never moved out." Robert said that Jane had epilepsy as a child and it affected her relationships with other children. He alluded to Jane's having other medical and psychological problems as well that might explain why she was living with her mother at forty-three, but he made it clear he was not going to explain it to me. Karen, on the other hand, seemed quite open about it as we sat in her kitchen a month later and talked about her family. She told me that Jane was born with a cleft palate and had gone through many operations. Despite the difference in their willingness to discuss Jane, both Karen and Robert accept that their sister cannot or will not help them in caring for their mother. Karen offered her understanding of why Jane is not interested in caring for her mother.

Jane says that Mom's been yelling at her all her life. I don't remember that. I slept all the time as a child, I don't know why. When my mom is really bad she's really abusive. Jane says: "I'm used to this, she's yelled at me all my life."

Neither Robert nor Karen expressed any disappointment that Jane is not an equal partner in the process of caring for their mother. Their acceptance of Jane's refusal to participate in caring for their mother seems to be based on her traditional role in the family. She had medical issues, and so they seem to have learned not to expect anything from her. Indeed, this seems to have had secondary benefits for Jane. For example, although Jane is a college graduate and has a good job, Robert told me that he and Karen will give her the house that she shared with her mother when their mother dies.

Eventually, because of Robert's prodding, Karen agreed to put her mother in a nursing home. Before that, Robert told me he was afraid Karen was going to have a nervous breakdown because of the pressure of caring for her mother, her guilt about putting her in a nursing home and her responsibility for her sick husband.

Karen was cleaning my mother's house and taking her to doctors and doing everything she could. It was overburdening her. She has two kids and a sick husband.

Once Karen told Robert how overburdened she felt, the three siblings were able to share their experience of how difficult it was to deal with their mother. Before they put her in a nursing home, she needed twenty-four-hour care, but wanted to be at home, yet complained that there were too many people in the house. At that time Robert told me about how difficult it was to deal with his mother:

She's refusing help. We got someone from the Visiting Nurses Association aside from the nurse, but my mother started arguing by the second day. We can't get through to her that she's not helping herself. And if she goes into a nursing home, she'll probably not talk to anyone. But picking her up off the floor at 3 a.m. kills me. I'm a night person and I've only gone to bed at 2 a.m. and then I have to get up and go over there because she's fallen. It's difficult when someone just won't see what's right for them. The three of us got together and I said we just have to deal with the fact that we may have to force her to go into a nursing home.

Karen said that Robert didn't realize how much caregiving she had been doing. After her hospital stay, when it was clear that twenty-four-hour care was necessary, it was Robert that insisted that they had to put their mother in a nursing home despite her protestations.

These three siblings grew up so distant from one another, each trying to deal in his or her own way with a dying father and an overburdened mother, and they may never be emotional intimates. But the experience of caring for their mother brought them closer together. Robert says:

> The three of us have meetings now to talk about my mother. Before that we rarely saw one another and never got together with the three of us. I hope Karen gets over this and learns. She's got in-laws and her husband has only one brother, who is like my middle sister—pretty self-centered. Caring for her in-laws will fall on Karen, and knowing her she will feel the responsibility to do something.

Brothers and sisters draw on cultural definitions of gender that associate women with family work regardless of whether they are also employed outside the home. In most families in which there is a son and a daughter, gender is used as a taken-for-granted way to assign tasks.[17]

But that alone does not explain why Karen had so much trouble setting limits on her caregiving and why she did not turn to her sister and brother for help until she was desperate and felt out of control. That is not simply a function of gender, but the specific psychodynamic constellation in her family. Karen's father was very sick during her childhood;

her sister Jane had serious physical and emotional problems; and her mother was working to support the family and caring for her husband. Robert might have taken up the slack and been a nurturer to Karen, but he didn't. He turned away from the intense family problems and put his energy into school and theater productions. Instead of the children developing a support system for one another, they each existed in an isolated state, each developing their own adaptive strategies—cleaning for Karen, theater for Robert and being sick for Jane.

SIBLING RELATIONSHIPS can never be separate from the relationship to the parents. Hence, working out relationships among siblings involves working out feelings about parents as well. Sibling relationships occur in the context of a "family script" involving a complex set of relationships between each child and each parent and each child in relation to the other children and each parent.

Mutuality among adult siblings depends on feeling securely separate, which is based on having basic needs met early. Mutuality also means being able to see the other person as separate and having needs that are different from yours. It involves being able to feel that you are similar in certain ways, but different in others; it involves offering support and compassion, but not unquestioning loyalty. Mutuality allows for closeness that is not exclusive; it leaves room for other significant emotional relationships. If siblings had to band together because of a lack of parental involvement or they were alienated and polarized because of parental favoritism, mutuality is difficult to attain. In both cases, the identities of siblings remain entangled. Whether you remain tied to your brothers and sisters, or separate from them in ways that can never be bridged, the lifelong quest for a secure personal identity is inextricably woven into that of your brother or sister.

Robert, Karen and Jane did not get their own individual needs met enough to develop mutuality as children. Each one was too needy. Each one developed some way of trying to get their needs met. Now, with the crisis of their mother's illness, they are talking to one another on a regular basis. For the first time in their lives, these three siblings are sharing their experiences of their mother. They are beginning to partially identify with one another in a way that they were not able to as children, and they are developing mutuality which will benefit them all.

Part III

ETHNICITY
AND GENDER

Chapter Six

CULTURAL SCRIPTS
FOR CAREGIVERS

> Where I come from, in the islands—Jamaica—this is
> what you do. A mother has a daughter to take care of her
> when she gets old. This is our role; we grow up this way.

IN PREVIOUS CHAPTERS I have talked about the effects of
psychological and family dynamics on caregiving. However,
those dynamics play out within a social and cultural context.
The priority we give to our own needs as compared to our
children's or parents' needs is a combination of cultural and
psychological factors. Just as there are cultural scripts for
motherhood, there are cultural scripts for caregiving.

Though there is never a perfect correspondence between
individual behavior and cultural prescriptions for how and
what should take place, the script is like a map that guides
most people's choices.[1] Even if we don't follow the cultural
prescription, it impinges upon us. We feel we *should* be behaving in a particular way or we might imagine that other
people in our cultural group are critical of our choices—and

they *might* be. The interaction between the cultural and psychological scripts results in the particular constellation of caregiving in each family.

The dominant American cultural script for caregiving is that *a daughter* takes primary responsibility for caring for elderly parents.[2] Middle-aged daughters represent 77 percent of the children providing care for elderly parents.[3] However, in Chinese and Indian families the oldest son has primary responsibility for caring for his parents, though his wife does the work. In rural Ireland in the nineteenth century, when the eldest son inherited the family farm, the wife of the son who was going to inherit the farm was expected to look after her parents-in-law. But in urban America, women of Irish ancestry are expected to look after their own parents. Since Irish elderly are more likely to be born in the United States than Chinese elderly, for example, the cultural expectations of women of Irish ancestry are more congruous with those of the dominant American culture in contrast with women of Chinese ancestry.[4]

To some degree, the process of caregiver selection transcends cultural differences. Cultural values mediate the process primarily with respect to the gender of the child expected to assume the primary *responsibility*. Nevertheless it is usually a female who will take the primary caregiver role—either a daughter or a daughter-in-law.

Cultural differences not only affect *who* is deemed responsible for caring for elderly parents, but also *how*. For example, Latino-American and Caribbean-American caregivers tend to reject the idea of nursing homes—not just for financial reasons, but for moral reasons. They often feel that their parents *should* live with them and they should take care of them regardless of how they *feel* about them. During the waves of migration in the 1950s and '60s, Caribbean parents often migrated to the United States or to England without their children—leaving them behind with relatives for as long as five years. Despite their having been left behind, most of these now middle-aged daughters completely accept their role as caregiver to their aging parents and often care for the mother substitutes (that is, grandmothers, aunts, older sisters or cousins) who filled in while their mothers worked in the United States or England.

Italian-Americans also tend to reject institutional help and feel that they should personally care for their elderly parents even if they are incontinent and suffering from dementia. On the other hand, non-Orthodox Jews tend to feel that they have responsibility to see that their parents are cared for—but they don't necessarily have to *do it*.

The reality of different cultural scripts becomes clear when we look at the living situations of elderly members of different ethnic groups. For example, 28 percent of all Americans over sixty-five live alone, but only 12.9 percent of Asian-Americans and 18.2 percent of Latinos do. In contrast, 29.4 percent of non-Latino blacks over sixty-five live alone. Four percent of all Americans over sixty-five live with a child, but 22 percent of Asian-Americans do because of their strong feelings about honoring their parents. Almost 5 percent of the American population over sixty-five is institutionalized, but only 2.4 percent of the Latino elderly and 1.5 percent of Asians are. Asians, Latinos and blacks have strong cultural beliefs about family obligations and preferred living

arrangements—they are much more likely to live with a de-
mented parent than a white caregiver.[5]

At a recent conference, Ron Adelman, the cochief of the
Division of Geriatric Medicine and Gerontology at the Weill
Medical College of Cornell University, got a warm welcome
from the gathering of social workers who had come to a
panel titled "Can My Eighties Be Like My Fifties?" at the
New York Academy of Medicine. Ron is a warm man who
spoke about the need to train young physicians to speak to
their elderly patients when they had a question rather than
turning to their children as if the elderly person was invisi-
ble. He told a story about a patient he knew so well that he
could tell that the patient had an infection because he was
behaving differently in his office.

Then Ron told a story about his own father. When he lay
in the hospital wanting to die, he said to his son: "Ron, don't
do anything to help me that could get you in trouble." I'm
not sure if he had tears in his eyes or if I was projecting because I had tears in my eyes. What a caring thing for his father to say to him; he wanted to protect his son to the very
end. It was such a contrast to my father's words to me when
he was dying: "Take care of your mother." I thought to myself that probably much of the reason Ron is such a caring
doctor is because he had such a caring father. That must be
why he feels so empathetic toward elderly people. Yet even
though his father was so concerned with Ron's happiness
and my father was not concerned with mine, we share the
same cultural script. We were brought up with the expectation that when our parents got older, we would make sure
they got the care they needed. But we never considered hav-

ing them live with us. That is something we identify with the first generation of immigration from Europe. My grandmother lived with my aunt Hannah, but Hannah's children never considered the possibility of her living with them.

After Ron spoke, Michael Diaz, professor of medicine at Mount Sinai Medical Center, introduced himself. "Hi, I'm Mike," he said, immediately making it clear that he did not want to pull rank on a roomful of social workers. Mike told us that he was born in Puerto Rico and had come to East Harlem with his parents as a baby. He talked about how elderly Hispanic and black people come to the doctor's office with one or more family members. He seemed to be chiding those of us (like me) who sent an aide to the doctor's office with one of our parents when it was an inconvenient time for us—or worse yet let the parent go alone. He said that white doctors didn't even have enough chairs in their waiting rooms for relatives because they expect black and Hispanic families to behave like their own.

Mike takes pride in being Puerto Rican. He uses Spanish intermittently in his talk the way Jewish doctors sometimes use Yiddish expressions. He proudly told us that when he got married and he and his wife bought a house, they bought one that had an extra floor for the express purpose of having it available for their parents to live with them when they got older—and, indeed, his parents did live with him.

Here were two "good sons." Each one spoke lovingly of his parents. Each one feels great empathy for elderly people. Yet one, the Jewish doctor, never dreamed of having his parents live with him; while the other, a Puerto Rican doctor, would never have thought of his parents *not* living with him.

Even when the social class is the same (they are both doctors), having come from different ethnic backgrounds, their cultural scripts are different.

While it is true that the dominant American script for caregiving is that *a daughter* is supposed to take primary responsibility for caring for elderly parents, if there is no daughter, a son may end up being the caregiver—particularly if he is an only child or if he is Hispanic or Italian.

AN ITALIAN SON

At sixty-six years old, Vinny is a widower taking care of his ninety-four-year-old father. Vinny feels that he has no choice; he feels this is what he's "supposed" to do. He and his wife took care of her mother for eighteen years before she died at ninety-four.

> She came to live with us when I was forty-one, twenty-five years ago. We never went on vacation. We went out sometimes because my son lived upstairs, but we couldn't go away for any length of time.

According to Vinny's cultural script, like Mike Diaz's, elderly parents live with their children and it doesn't matter how the children feel about it or what condition the parents are in. Vinny described his mother-in-law's condition:

> We had to put a rope from her bedroom to the bathroom because she would stray. She'd go to the bathroom and end up in our bedroom turning the light on in the middle of the night.

"Did she have Alzheimer's?" I asked. Vinny didn't know. They never took her to a neurologist to find out. It didn't matter. Whatever it was, they would take care of her. His mother-in-law died in 1990 and then, in 1994, Vinny's mother died. "My father has macular degeneration. So he couldn't live alone, he had to come and live with us." Vinny could see no other options. In reality he had several choices: He could have found an assisted living facility for his father; he could have hired a visiting nurse to come to his house; or he could have insisted that his brother take more responsibility for his father.

"How did you feel about your father coming to live with you?" I asked.

"I had no choice, what could I do?"

My question reflects my cultural script: How you *feel* is a major consideration in making decisions. Vinny's answer ignores the issue of how he felt about it. It reflects the combination of his cultural script and his depression. In reality, Vinny had several choices, but he could not consider them. He had an internalized cultural script for what "a good son," an *Italian* son, is supposed to do, but he also has an insecure attachment to his father. He needs his father's approval and he cannot tolerate being separate from him. That would involve tolerating his father's anger and disappointment that Vinny will not give up his life for him. Vinny complains:

He can't see and he depends on me for everything. But it's really hard. Like I could just have a cup of coffee and run out the door. But he wants breakfast and so I have to make him this big breakfast every morning. I met a woman, but

I can never see her. Taking care of my father is holding me back. I don't have a life. When I walk out of the house I feel guilty that he's alone. It's a lousy feeling that the only way out of it is my father dying.

I asked Vinny if he has thought about hiring some help. He said that he can't get an aide paid for by the state because his father has too much money. He owns too many houses—four of them. I asked him if he considered the possibility of paying for help. But he said that's impossible because his father won't spend the money. To underscore the point, he told me:

I go to Arizona with my father for the winter. But all I do is work when I get there. His houses need a lot of work and next to his house he bought this piece of property and planted this big garden. We call it a "Guinea garden." He's got lemon trees, olive trees, all kinds of trees, but they all have to be taken care of. When I went there with my wife she said: "You can't do this. This is ridiculous. You're retired."

Vinny's father's refusal to spend money keeps Vinny taking care of him. For example, Vinny recounted that he wanted to get him a Med Alert. He explained that his father could wear it around his neck so that Vinny would feel comfortable going out and leaving him alone. When Vinny explained this to his father he said: "How much is it?" Vinny told him the price and he said: "I don't need that." So Vinny feels he cannot leave his father alone. At sixty-six Vinny still feels that whatever his father says goes. He cannot stand up to his father or even his older brother.

Vinny's brother, Sal, is three and a half years older. Vinny said that Sal doesn't offer to help.

> Even when my wife was sick and I was caring for my wife *and* my father, Sal never offered to take my father. Everybody says, Why don't you tell your brother that you each have to take your father for six months? I can't do it. My father would feel like I was throwing him out.

Although Sal does not participate in the care of his father, it is Sal who has power of attorney. Vinny explained: "We're Italians—he's the oldest brother, so he has the authority."

Vinny is a good example of the interaction between cultural and psychological scripts. He is Italian, but he is also clinically depressed. He feels powerless and hopeless. He feels guilty because his only relief will come when his father dies. His normal activities are constricted by the kind of caregiving he feels obligated to perform. He is engulfed by his father's needs and demands and cannot separate enough to have a relationship with a woman. Since he is a retired widower, caring for his father is his only role and has probably intensified his feeling like a little boy who has to "obey" his father and older brother. His older brother is also Italian and, of course, has the same controlling and demanding father. But Sal seems to have been able to separate more. He does not need to show his father what a good son he is—perhaps because he feels more secure in his attachment to his father.

Vinny's brother seems to have cast off his responsibility as the older son in an Italian family. On the other hand, Vinny feels hog-tied by his cultural script. How can he have a life that is separate from his father without discarding heartfelt traditions? Vinny has to set limits so that he is able to take care of himself, and his father gets the care he needs. Of course, the care he *needs* is not necessarily the same as the care he *wants*. Once he makes that distinction, Vinny will have to tolerate his father's complaints and accept that his father may not appreciate him, even though he is striving to do the right thing.

AN AFRICAN-AMERICAN DAUGHTER

Traditionally, studies of ethnicity showed that elderly non-Hispanic blacks were less likely to be in nursing homes than non-Hispanic white elderly. However, the trend has been toward convergence in the last thirty years.[6] In 1990, 3.1 percent of black (non-Hispanic) Americans over sixty-five were institutionalized as compared to 3.3 percent of non-Hispanic whites. In 2000, 5.4 percent of non-Hispanic blacks over sixty-five lived in institutions. Indeed, the percentage of blacks over sixty-five in institutions was actually slightly higher than the percent of white (non-Hispanic) Americans. A recent study argues that young blacks have strong ideals of filial obligation and do not generally want to put their kin in nursing homes. Black caregivers report that they were brought up with the expectation of becoming caregivers—many have been caregivers from an early age. The authors of a study of black caregivers in Ohio point out that there is a "culture of caring."[7] Sixty-two percent of black nursing home residents as compared to 23.2 percent of other residents, for example, lived with children before entering nursing homes. In other words, living with children seems to be part of an elderly black person's trajectory into a nursing home much more commonly than it is for white elderly. However, the higher levels of impairment of the black elders may often make it impossible for their children to care for them at home despite their commitment to do so. Sally is trying to keep her mother out of a nursing home despite the high personal cost to her and her children and the protestations of her siblings.

Sally called the Senior Day Care Center to find out if I was coming to interview caregivers. She wanted to make sure that I would interview her. I called to tell her that I had reached my quota of interviews, but she pleaded with me. I told her I could only fit her in early on Saturday morning. She said that was fine; she wanted to talk to me. I wondered why she was so eager to tell me her story. When I arrived at the center, at 8 a.m., Sally was waiting for me. She is an attractive African-American woman wearing a stylish black suit. She greets me warmly as I come in apologizing for being a few minutes late because I got lost. She's eager to talk and seems excited about our interview.

She is a forty-one-year-old divorced mother of four. Her husband left her five years ago. She has three daughters, seven, ten, and fourteen years old and a nineteen-year-old son. Her ten-year-old daughter has cerebral palsy. When Sally's mother's friends called her and told her that her mother was incontinent and could not take care of herself, Sally took the three-hour drive to check on her. Her mother wasn't taking her medicines because she couldn't remember what to take or when. Initially, Sally hoped she could keep her mother in her apartment and visit her a couple of days a week. However, when Sally came back after each visit, her mother called every few minutes to ask her something.

Finally, Sally's five brothers and sisters decided their mother could no longer live alone. Sally describes her mother as a sixty-three-year-old in the body of an eighty-year-old. She has kidney failure as a result of diabetes, so she is required to be on dialysis three days each week, and her right leg has been amputated. She had a stroke and has dementia. Sally says her siblings all pointed to her as the one who should take care of her mother because she's not married and she is a nurse. They did not seem to consider that she is a working single mother with four children, one of whom is disabled.

> To be honest I really didn't want to take care of my mother. I was going through a divorce and it was too much. I was overwhelmed. But it's always been like that all my life. I was the one they called "the workhorse." They knew I didn't want my mom in a nursing home and if that was the alternative I would do it. My mom got really sick and my brother went to get her and just dropped her off at my house!

Sally was working 11 a.m. to 7 p.m. as well as caring for her children when her mother arrived at her doorstep. "It was unbelievable." Sally had not lived with her mother since she left home at seventeen to go to the state college. Since Sally's mother had never been willing to help care for her grandchildren, Sally's children did not know their grandmother very well. Her three daughters share a room and her son has a room so Sally gave her mother her bedroom.

> During that time my younger sister took my mom on weekends, but she and my mother never got along. My sis-

ter already had marital problems before my mother arrived, but then my mother was incontinent and would shit all over the house and walk around naked in front of my brother-in-law. My sister would call and tell me she was going to throw my mother out the window. I would come to the rescue. But after a while I just couldn't do it anymore. I'd go over to their house and my sister and brother-in-law were fighting and I'd have to clean my mother and get her dressed and take her home with me.

Why was Sally willing to take on the added responsibility of caring for her mother when she was already overwhelmed by her husband leaving her to support and care for four children? She was not motivated by the hope of mutual assistance because her mother had never cared for her grandchildren when she was well and was now unable to help in any way. Sally was not motivated by love and respect. She did not feel that she owed her mother anything. I think the answer is in Sally's identification as the "hero" of the family.

Sally's mother and father separated when she was twelve—her mother took the children and left. Sally says her father didn't pay child support so her mom cleaned schools and people's houses. Sally says she was the only one who could sit down and talk to her father. He drank and was abusive to her mother and the children. He worked in the steel mills and was often laid off. He traveled to different places to get work. She recalls watching him waiting for his check to come.

He smoked and he would smoke while he was eating. Sometimes he didn't finish eating and he put his plate in the refrigerator and he dropped ashes in the plate. Then he'd come home at 2 a.m. and wake us all up and line us up and scream that one of us is doing voodoo on him and we put ashes in his food. He'd beat us. Then we went to sleep and woke up the next morning and went to school. We knew it was going to happen. Then he'd give us "times off." He said our bottoms were getting too used to it so he'd give us "times off." Then it would start again.

I asked Sally if her father was drunk when he did this and she said no, she thinks he was psychotic.

He used to do this thing we called "fighting with the devil." My dad would go to the graveyard and bring dirt back to the house. He'd be yelling and hitting himself. When we got out of school, we knew we better have the house clean. We knew he'd beat us. We couldn't hear his car coming, hear his steps. We knew we had to get out of his way. If he were happy in the morning, he'd be abusive in the evening. If he were abusive in the evening, he'd be happy in the morning.

I asked Sally, "What did your mother do?" Her reply was that her mother did nothing. In fact, her father sexually abused her and her sister Lilly. She said he would make excuses to drive her somewhere and sexually abuse her in the car. She described her fantasy of screaming at the people passing by on the street: "Help me, help me." But she was silent.

She feels that her mother did not know he was abusing her, but she feels her mother knew he was abusing her sister.

My mother was very harsh with my younger sister. She was my father's favorite and my mother hated her. She would take an extension cord when Lilly was in the bath and hit her with it in the tub. Or other times my father was away and we'd all be scared and run to my mother's bedroom and she'd make Lilly leave and go upstairs alone. Lilly would be crying and yelling.

Sally said that once her sister showed her a story in the newspaper about a girl who accused her father of sexually abusing her and her mother threw her out of the house. They both smiled knowingly—they felt their mother would do the same thing.

Considering that her mother did not protect her from her father and was abusive toward her younger sister, it is hard to understand how it came to pass that Sally's mother lived with her for almost a year until Sally was able to put her mother in a low-income senior citizen apartment complex.

As I listened to Sally's story about her mother coming to stay with her, I thought to myself that it sounded like she was on the brink of a major depression during that time. She was suffering from chronic fatigue, anger and frustration. But then Sally's face changed. The anger and frustration were gone. To my surprise, she said:

I believe it was God that made a great difference. I was resistant to taking care of my mom. I respected her as my mom, but never had any deep love for her. But when I began to take care of her something in me began to happen. What has happened is that taking care of her made me start to [her face beaming] *fall in love with her.* I began to see things in her the way I see things in my children. All my energies turned to trying to make her survive and have a quality life. When she first came to my house I got a prognosis of two years and it's been three years.

As for so many African-American caregivers, her religious belief has been a major support for Sally. She feels a sense of personal enrichment and character building as a result of caring for her mother. Sally explained that she went to college to become a nurse, but she never graduated; she got pregnant and dropped out. Her mother was very disappointed in her.

So when my mother was at her worst, refusing to eat and wanting to die after her leg was amputated, I told her I was going to go back to school and she had to eat so that she could see me walk across the stage and get my diploma. My mother began to eat again. Last year I walked across the stage and she was there. That was the happiest moment of my life. It's made me a better person.

Sally went on to explain that: "This is life. Things happen and they don't happen the way we want, but then you have to be more organized." Sally had to deal with her mother's surgeries, her daughter's seizures and having finals all at the same time! To my amazement, she said:

It made me know what true love was all about. I never felt love for her, but when she was so tired and I would say: "Mom I need you to help, stand up." I could see her trying so hard. She would cry out for me: "Sally, Sally." It did something to me. I felt it's not all about me. You have to make sacrifices—I think my character has improved. I look at life differently.

Whereas Vinny's caregiving has led to a constriction of his social life and normal activities—living with his father has made him feel less and less like a man and more and more like a boy—Sally's caregiving has enhanced her sense of competence. It has increased her feeling of mastery and her self-esteem. She went back to finish college while caring for her mother. She was able to get low-cost housing for her mother and found a center where her mother can be cared for during the day. Sally goes to her mother's house every morning before she goes to work to wake her up, take her vital signs, give her medicine and get her dressed and ready to take the van to the day-care center. Then after work, Sally meets her mom at the van and stays for several hours. I asked her how she manages this with four children at home. Sally reassured me that she has raised them to take care of themselves. She told me that she prepares their meals ahead of time, but in an emergency her fourteen-year-old daughter and nineteen-year-old son know how to prepare meals. She casually explained that they have a pager so that if her ten-year-old daughter has a seizure, one of the older children pages her. Her sisters and brothers took a vote and decided their mother should be put in a nursing home, but Sally has the power of attorney and she refuses to do it.

Caring for her mother makes her feel like a hero—she is single-handedly saving her mother, and the gratification of that seems to outweigh the costs. Part of me is in awe of Sally. She has been able to turn her caregiving into a growth-promoting, transformative experience. But then, there is another part of me that has my own cultural script. My script says: Caring for your children takes precedence over caring for your parents. Clearly, her children are paying a price for their mother's heroism. Sally's two older children are left to care for themselves and their two younger sisters, one of whom is disabled. That does not seem to cause Sally any conflict. Perhaps this is due to her cultural script for mothering. Like so many African-American mothers, Sally feels that she needs to prepare her children to take care of themselves. Or perhaps it has more to do with her personal psychological script—her insecure attachment to her mother makes her need to feel close to her mother and appreciated by her. Wanting to be close to and appreciated by your mother can be a positive thing, but for Sally it is a driving force that keeps her focused so intensely on her mother that her children's needs become incidental. Hence, she has reproduced the same dynamic in the next generation. Her two older children are "heroes" in the making. They are doing the mothering while their mother is being a "good daughter."

A PUERTO RICAN DAUGHTER

Although the Latino population is composed of many diverse subgroups, extended family plays a salient role for all of them. Respect for elders is paramount, so it is no surprise that elderly Latinos are more likely to live with their children than in any other ethnic group.[8] While dementia greatly increases the chances that a non-Latino white elder will be put in a nursing home, Latino caregivers are less disturbed by memory loss and the inability to communicate.

Maria is a fifty-one-year-old single professor. Her seventy-nine-year-old mother has lived with her for the last six years, beginning soon after she was diagnosed with Alzheimer's disease. When Maria greeted me and escorted me into her office, she excused herself for a minute before we began our interview. When she returned Maria was beaming and handed me a picture of her mother wearing a graduation cap. The caption under her name said "Doctor of Philosophy, *honoris causa.*" Although her mother cannot speak or move, Maria was eager to have me meet her and gave me the picture because the venue for the interview was changed from her house to her office and I would not get to meet her.

Maria explained that her mother, Hortensia, was a well-educated woman. Hortensia's father was the mayor of their town and a political activist. When he had a stroke, Hortensia dropped out of college to care for him because she was the eldest daughter in the family and felt it was her obligation. Maria's father, on the other hand, was one of seventeen children born on a farm and only had an eighth-grade education. Indeed, her parents first met when her mother was teaching her father, Carlos, to speak English as a second language in preparation for his family moving to the mainland. Maria believes Hortensia saw Carlos as someone who would offer her adventure and take her away from her caregiving role with her father, but ironically she ended up taking care of Carlos—first by supporting his driving need to prove himself worthy of her and later by caring for him when he became ill.

Maria's parents married and moved to the South Bronx with his family in 1947. Maria says that although her mother loved her father, marrying a man of a lower social class had lifelong consequences for her. Her family remained in Puerto Rico and her mother never approved of the marriage. While Hortensia was able to be a teacher in Puerto Rico, in New York she could not teach without a college degree. She worked as a seamstress in a factory doing piecework, while her husband worked in a bodega. Maria remembers that there was never enough money, but there was always food. Her father dreamed of owning his own bodega (which he eventually did) and becoming middle class. He was driven. Maria describes him as a hardworking but macho man who was very controlling. She feels that her mother's identity faded away. In fact, Maria has her own theory about the etiology of Alzheimer's based on her feelings about her parents. She believes that people who lose their sense of self because of a controlling spouse or parent are more likely to develop the disease. So although Maria speaks lovingly of her father, she sees her mother's marriage to him as tragic in some way—her mother was never the same. I wondered, as I listened to her theory of how living with a controlling person can lead to losing your self and your mind, if that might be related to Maria's choice to remain single.

At first Maria told me that she is the primary caregiver because her sister, Victoria, has lupus, but as we talked more Maria said that there are deeper reasons. She explained that her mother always favored her sister.

My mother always paid more attention to my sister. She had more needs. She was always sick and they never figured out what was wrong with her. She had headaches. She was tired.

Maria tried to be the opposite. She developed a strong persona, she tried to look tough and not need anything. Her father worked twelve to fifteen hours a day, seven days a week, and since her mother was also working, Maria was often left in the care of her older sister, Victoria. While Maria says that Victoria made lunch and loved to clean the house, she was not very nurturing. Nevertheless, Maria says:

A lot of people say my mother has advanced Alzheimer's, she can't walk or talk. Why don't you put her in a nursing home?

Maria feels they just don't understand. First, they don't understand that Puerto Rican daughters don't put their mothers in nursing homes—no matter how poorly they might function. Moreover, Maria says they don't know her mother and that she still is attached despite the Alzheimer's disease. But, I think what they don't understand is Maria's attachment to her mother. They don't understand the gratification that Maria gets from caring for her mother. For example, when I first met her at her office she told me about losing her briefcase the day before. It contained student papers, her Palm Pilot and other irreplaceable items. I could feel the anxiety well up in me at the idea of losing mine. She found the briefcase after several hours of panic, and she turned to her vacant mother and said: "You knew I'd find it didn't you?" And when her mother smiled, probably understanding nothing of what had gone on in the previous several hours, Maria felt filled up and loved. Here is the key to Maria's pleasure in caring for her mother despite all the sacrifices it entails—financial and career sacrifices, getting up in the middle of the night to clean or otherwise care for her, and giving up a social life to make dinner and feed her mother every night. Maria's mother is a "good mother." Maria projects on her all the loving, accepting feelings that she did not feel from her as a child. When she was a child her mother turned away from her to Victoria. But now her mother's smile warms her heart in a way that she always wanted. Her mother isn't cooking for her father or taking care of her sister. Her mother belongs to her. Her mother is always there for her. Maria says she was always jealous of the relationship between her mother and her sister because her sister got all the attention. But she is the good daughter. She always was a good daughter, but now she is *the* good daughter. Her mother needs her and she takes care of her.

> Alzheimer's, I wonder how much of a blessing it is sometimes. When I don't feel well, she can pick it up. When I'm in a really good mood, she can pick that up. I think there are pieces that she can pick up and I feel really good when I can read her.

Maria feels that her mother is attuned to her moods and feelings. Maria experiences her as loving and concerned. In that sense the Alzheimer's has been a blessing for Maria, if not her mother. Indeed, when her mother was diagnosed with Alzheimer's she told Maria that she knew Maria would bear the burden of caring for her. She said: "Eventually I will know nothing and you will know everything." She held Maria as she sobbed and told her she was sorry for what she would have to bear. Maria had borne the burden of not being the chosen favorite for her entire life. Only when her mother developed Alzheimer's did she fully appreciate Maria.

VINNY, Sally and Maria are caregivers who have followed their cultural scripts. But, not everyone does. For example, Latinos may be *more likely* to have their elderly parents live with them, but not all of them do. In addition, siblings who have the same cultural scripts respond to them in different ways. Sally's siblings, Vinny's brother and Maria's sister did not follow their cultural scripts. However, it is possible to negotiate beyond one's cultural script without rejecting it entirely. For example, my friend Susan, whom I described earlier has become fluent in Italian and traveled to Italy to trace her family's history; she teaches a course on Italian-American writers. Susan is an Italian-American daughter who decided not to have her mother live with her, but arranged things so that her mother could live in her own house, as she requested, and not go to a nursing home. Adhering to your cultural script need not be an all-or-nothing choice. Susan is proud of her traditions and does not want to turn away from her mother. However, insisting on adhering to a cultural script when it is destructive to self and family is a psychological issue.

Is it a psychological *problem* for Vinny, Sally and Maria to care for their elderly parents? Or are they doing what is expected of them in their cultural context? How do we evaluate cultural norms that are different from our own? Is it *right* to have your parents live with you and make sacrifices for them or is it *wrong*? I don't think it is either right or wrong. I think the degree to which Vinny has given up his own life to care for his father has made him depressed and therefore it is a problem. He does not find it gratifying to care for his father. He does not feel, as Sally does, that it has made him a more competent person or given him a greater sense of mastery. On the contrary, it has made him regress to feeling like a boy who has to do what his father wants no matter what. On the other hand, Sally has followed her cultural script and found a way to make caring for her mother a gratifying experience. *But* her gratification has sometimes come at the cost of neglecting her children. Therefore, from my perspective, it remains a problem.

Finally, Maria has found caring for her mother a gratifying experience. Although Latinos are the most likely group to live with their elderly parents and care for them, research has shown they experience a high level of stress from doing so. Feeling a sense of filial obligation and stress from fulfilling it seem to go hand in hand for Latinos. But this is not the case with Maria. She is doing what Latinas are expected to do and her family in Puerto Rico is very supportive of her. She is also getting something from her mother that she has always yearned for—she feels she is the special daughter and is finally closer to her mother than her sister is. Maria does not have children, so caring for her mother has not impacted them. She has never married, but feels that she would not have done so anyway for reasons that are probably related to her early relationship with her mother, but not to her caregiving. Therefore, in Maria's case, there seems to be a perfect fit between her cultural script and her psychological needs.

Chapter Seven

DAUGHTERS

> Do I love her? Yes, but not in the same way as those
> who say "I love my mother, I could never put her in a
> home." For loves are like people, each is different, and
> they are not just the same love which finds different
> objects to attach to.[1]

I FELT SO RELIEVED when I read Linda Grant's feelings
about her mother, quoted above; there are different kinds of
loving. It would be painful to feel that I don't love my
mother. No one wants to feel that. In some places, like Manhattan, many people have been in therapy and accept their
ambivalent feelings toward their parents. But in other places,
expressions of ambivalence are met with shock. People look
at you strangely if you don't visit your mother regularly or
talk frequently on the phone. I usually don't talk about my
mother in rural Connecticut where I have a weekend home
because, feeling so conflicted about her, talking to people
who don't express any ambivalence usually makes me feel
bad about myself. I ask myself: What's wrong with me that I
have so many angry feelings about my mother? So it was cu-

rious that when Patricia told me about her mother I didn't feel bad about myself. I felt jealous of her admiration for her mother; I felt envious of her awe. But I didn't feel bad about myself.

Patricia is fifty-five and her mother, Charlotte, died six years ago. She is a friend of the director of the senior center where I was interviewing caregivers in Columbus, Ohio, and heard about my study from her. She called to ask me if I would *please* interview her, even though her mother died six years ago, because she was eager to talk about her. I met Patricia at her office in a Columbus hospital where she is the director of the hospice program. She is an attractive blonde, very well dressed, warm and eager to talk. Crammed into a very small office with her employees right outside the door, Patricia cried throughout our interview—and so did I.

Patricia's mother, a double amputee, had breast cancer five years before she died and it recurred and spread the second time. She refused any further treatment and chose to have only palliative care. She remained at home throughout her illness and was up and about until three weeks before she died.

Patricia has an older sister and two younger brothers. She also has two stepsisters whose mother died before they were five. After her mother was diagnosed, although she did not have any symptoms for several months, the out-of-town siblings began visiting New Hampshire more often. Charlotte began having symptoms and became ill one day when Patricia was at the house on one of her three- or four-day shifts. Her mother went to bed that day and it was the beginning of a three-week bedside vigil. All six siblings gathered at her mother and stepfather's house. One brother came from California; her sister came from New Jersey; another sister came from Connecticut.

Patricia says they created their own hospice team at home. They made sure that someone was with her all the time. Patricia knew how to set up a hospice team because she had been working in a hospice program for thirteen years. She always felt her mother was very supportive of the kinds of things she was doing in hospice work, so it made good sense to her that her mother would choose to die that way. Her mother modeled what Patricia called "a beautiful death."

At the beginning of the first week, her mother directly discussed dying. But soon she didn't have the strength to talk. She could only whisper. She wrote everything down. She wrote logs about what she wanted to say. Patricia speaks in an awestruck tone about how her mother dealt with her death. She says:

> She brought each of us in to ask what we wanted of her belongings. For example, I always wanted her Wedgwood. She did this for each of her children. Then she did it for each of her grandchildren. She had one grandchild who was getting married. She talked to him about the woman he was marrying. She had another grandson who was college age. She talked to him about how he felt about different schools. She talked to a third grandson about the trip he just took to Africa. When she was talking to him she was on a respirator and she asked him to trace the trip on the map for her. She didn't want to miss anything.

Charlotte was able to be open and generous while she was dying. Patricia went on appreciatively about her mother:

Another day she asked to see each of the grandchildren again because she wanted to give them some direction. She told my son, in writing, he should stop using the word "like." She wrote that a thing "is" or "is not," it's not "like." He asked her if the bird at the feeder outside the window was a chickadee or a nut hen. She drew the beak of each one to illustrate the difference. She had so much knowledge and education and she wanted to share it to the end.

I was struck by how much Patricia respected and admired her mother. She felt she and her children could learn important things from her mother and that her mother was full of those important things—from grammar to a knowledge of birds to how to die. She admired the way her mother lived her life and the way she went about dying. I felt jealous of the twinkle in Patricia's eyes when she told me about her. I felt jealous of Patricia for having a mother whom she *wanted to be like*. She viewed her mother as strong and wise, but also brave. She began telling me how much suffering her mother overcame.

Patricia's father was a hematologist at a famous cancer hospital. At the top of his field and outwardly upstanding, he had a secret life. He was a bigamist—he married another woman because she was pregnant. He told Charlotte when Patricia was in the fifth grade. Her mother was devastated and decided to leave him and move to her parents' house in New Hampshire. Patricia's father drove the four children to the house, and her mother arrived soon afterward with Ethel, the babysitter. The same day they arrived, Patricia's grandmother had a stroke while driving with three of her grandchildren. Her grandmother died with Patricia's brothers and sister in the backseat. When Charlotte arrived eager to be comforted by her mother, she found out her mother was dead. Not surprisingly, she went into a major depression. She didn't get out of bed for over a year. She spoke to her psychiatrist in New York twice a week on the phone. Ethel took care of the children. Eventually, Charlotte got out of bed and went to secretarial school. She worked for a friend of the family who ran a tourism journal.

Then she started having trouble with her back and had a back operation. That was the beginning of another terrible experience.

She had a rare back disease that was first diagnosed when she was forty. They were never sure what it came from. They thought it might have been that she had a spinal during the delivery of one of her children that was not completely sterile. It was an inflammation around the spinal cord. She had braces on her legs and then used a cane and then, finally, when her legs were amputated, a wheelchair. She stopped walking when she was fifty. She had been a tall, athletic woman—a tennis player. The first two years in the wheelchair she was very depressed, but eventually she adjusted and got around fine. At the end, she would get into the car and fold up her wheelchair by herself.

Charlotte modeled the ability to experience great pain and still be able to be autonomous and separate. She did not try to get her children to take care of her when she could not walk—she folded up the wheelchair and put it in the car. She valued doing things on her own as long as she was able.

Patricia wasn't with her mother when she died. She had left two days before. She doesn't seem to feel any guilt about it. Rather, she explains to me that her siblings who were there had never experienced death before. They all held hands and held their mother's hands when she died. She explains it as if her mother was so powerful that she planned it that way—another gift to her children.

> It's so amazing that my mother chose to die with the children who didn't know what it was like. She wanted to show them what a beautiful death could be like and not to be scared. We often run away from people who are dying because it's so frightening and she really shared with them a beautiful death. It was a wonderful experience for my brothers and sisters. They weren't scared. They didn't want to run away.

Physical caregiving and/or intimate conversations with an elderly mother evoke a complex array of feelings. For Patricia, caring for her mother in the last weeks of her life made her feel closer to and more admiring of her. Patricia said her mother taught her about dying—let her know how it felt as she went through it.

In contrast to Patricia, I cannot identify with my mother's emotional and intellectual experience of aging because we never talked about our internal experiences. Our conversations were, and are, limited to day-to-day experiences— where did you go; what did you do; how much did it cost? We have never talked about how anything *feels*.

Although I don't identify with my mother's feelings and I don't see her as a role model, I do identify with her physi-

cally. I look like her and I am built like her. My body is changing as hers did. I have that stomach that sticks out a bit and
increasing numbers of brown spots on my face and hands.
Arthritis and bunions do not mangle my hands and feet, but
I have bursitis in my left arm and many mornings I have
trouble hooking my bra, just like my mother does. I have
wrinkles on my face in the same places as she did at my age
and I know they will deepen into the crevices she has around
her lips and chin. Patricia bathed her mother and helped her
go to the bathroom and was not repulsed by her mother's
legless body. But I have different feelings. Unlike Patricia, I
have spent my life trying to be different than my mother.
While Patricia admired her mother and wanted to be like her,
I hate myself for all the ways that I am like her.

IT'S 91 DEGREES and I am sweating from walking one
block from my air-conditioned car to Harbor View—my
mother's assisted living facility. It's in Sheepshead Bay in
Brooklyn and there's always a breeze, but nevertheless I'm
sweating. I'm planning to take my mother for our usual walk
over to the ice cream store where we empty her purse of the
cookie-crusted pennies she collects and use them to buy her
a chocolate Häagen-Dazs pop. My mother loves them. They
have dark chocolate outside and milk chocolate ice cream inside. The Korean storeowner impatiently waits each time I
count out all the pennies and wipe the cookie crumbs off.
After that I'm looking forward to going on a new adventure—finding the Home Depot in Brooklyn. It's in a part of
Brooklyn that I don't know and I've left plenty of time for
getting lost. I'm relishing the challenge.

When I find her in the large room where most of the elderly residents spend their day, she is sitting in her usual spot wearing a black velvet jacket over a long-sleeved wool sweater and a wool skirt. "Mom, aren't you hot?" I exclaim. She's drinking hot tea! I kiss her hello and ask her if she'd rather go have chocolate ice cream and leave the tea. She excitedly agrees. I suggest she leave her jacket there since it's so hot outside. An aide takes the jacket and whispers in my ear: "She's put on some weight and she doesn't really have any summer clothes she can wear." I feel guilty. I was in Europe for two weeks and haven't seen my mother since she had her cataract operation three weeks ago. While I was away there was a terrible heat wave in New York. She must have been sweltering. Forget Home Depot. I take her shopping for summer clothes after we get the ice cream.

When we get to Loehmann's to buy her clothes, there's not much to choose from—it's the end of July. I realize, also, that I don't know her size anymore. She was a size 10 most of her life, but I don't know what she is now. It's easy to buy her tops—she needs a large. But I never bought slacks with her and I have no idea what size will work. So I choose all different sizes and we head for the dressing room. The dressing room is upstairs. We'll take the elevator. No, they're moving garbage on the elevator; we have to take the escalator. Oh, no, I feel worried about my mother getting on an escalator. She doesn't see well and I'm afraid she will fall. But we make it upstairs safely and head for the dressing room. Suddenly, I feel this panic. Is she wearing a bra? She hasn't been wearing a bra much in recent years. It's too hard for her to hook it in the back. It's an open dressing room. I hate Loehmann's dressing room; I'm always afraid I'll meet a pa-

tient when I'm in my underwear. But the prices are so cheap.
Thank God, today she's wearing a bra. I don't want to look at
her breasts, I don't like to see how they sag down and meet
her stomach. It's so upsetting when I take her to doctors and
they assume I'm going to go into the examination room with
her. How can I not go with her? How can I not help her get
undressed? But I don't want to see her undressed. When I
took her to the gynecologist and his assistant assumed I was
going into the examination room with her, I thought I might
pass out. I waited until the doctor came to examine her, po-
litely excused myself and left the room.

I don't want to think about my breasts sagging all the way
to my stomach. I like my breasts. I've always taken pride in
the fact that they don't sag. But my stomach reminds me of
my mother's when she was my age. I cover it up with Eileen
Fisher, but it's all there. Now she's all stomach. I don't want
to look at her naked stomach. I fast walk; I play tennis; I do
my time on the treadmill. I don't want to have that stomach.

The room is full of young Russian women with heavy ac-
cents and old Jewish women whose parents were born in
Russia. We find a spot along the room-size mirror to hang all
the clothes of different sizes that I've gathered. On one side
of us, two of the old Jewish women are having an intense
conversation about how one of them can't get her pants up.
She's standing there in her panty hose with a stomach even
larger than my mother's. I'm afraid to look at her. I don't
want to see what she looks like without her pants. Her friend
is telling her it's not worth buying the pants on sale if she has
to put in a zipper. That will cost more than the pants would
cost full price. But, she responds, I can't get *any* pants up.
Her friend agrees that is a problem.

On the other side of us there's a young Russian woman wearing a pair of thong underpants. I'm facing her exposed behind. An older woman is telling her what a beautiful body she has and isn't it amazing that she has a child and still looks like that. I feel stuck in the middle, literally. On the one side is the body I'm afraid of having and on the other side is the body I never had!

It's time to try on the size 14 pants. My mother doesn't wear any underpants under her panty hose and I don't want to see her pubic hair. There's not much though and it's gray so it's kind of hard to see. It looks like she has none. I don't want to look closely to see if the hair's gray or gone. It's the same feeling as when I look at someone who is missing a limb and I can see the stump. It's a shock. I want to turn away. I've often wondered what that response is about.

The saleslady is Russian. She tells me it's pretty stupid to try those pants on. Don't I know my mother needs "petite"? Look how short she is! What a dope. I didn't think about petite. I sit my mother down and assure her I'll be back in a few minutes with some petite pants. I take the pile of wrong sizes out to the reject pile and set off to find the petite section. When I return, my mother is smiling and she's enjoying the banter in the dressing room. I help her step into each leg and pull up the pants. Bingo! We've got a light pair of pants and four sleeveless tops picked out for her. I have to help her put the wool skirt and long-sleeved sweater back on, but I console myself with the idea that in a little while I'll get her back to Harbor View and I'll get her out of that wool outfit and into something cool.

My mother is delighted when she changes into her cool new clothes. I feel like a good daughter. Now I can go to Home Depot.

At seventy-five, Lillian Rubin, sociologist and psychoanalyst, writes in her memoir, *Tangled Lives,* that she has also spent her life trying not to be like her mother. If you have an overly ambivalent relationship with your mother, you identify with her in a way that is not fully digested. Psychoanalysts call this type of identification an "introject." It is a part of you that is "not you"—a hated part of your self. When it emerges from you it feels excruciating.

A few days ago my younger son, Jason, twenty years old, sat down and told me that I make him feel guilty about spending money. He said every time I hand my charge card to a salesperson I have a grimace on my face. He told me that I still feel like I'm a poor kid from Brooklyn while the reality is that I'm an upper-middle-class professional woman from Manhattan. I cried. I felt pained. He is right.

Jason went on to say that I always use money as a reason for things—even when he knows that it's not about money. For example, there has been tension in our house for weeks because my husband and I want Jason to work as many weeks as possible during the summer before he goes off to Oxford for his junior year abroad. He has eighteen weeks off between finishing his sophomore year and going to Oxford. We want him to have money to travel while he is there. But, says Jason, we could give him enough money to travel. It is not that we *can't afford* to give him the money to travel while he is there. And, Jason goes on, why isn't working twelve weeks enough? Why do we insist he has to work sixteen weeks and only have two weeks off? "Why don't you talk about the real issue instead of making the issue money?" asks my very wise young son.

What *is* the real issue? What past reality am I bringing to this situation with my son? I remember the summer, as I described in the introduction, when I was five or six years old and my mother wouldn't buy me ice cream.

Oh God, am I doing the same thing to my son that my mother did to me? Am I saying: "You can't have six weeks of sleeping late and not working"? I even blurted out to him at one point: "*I* don't have six weeks' vacation." What nerve, I was telling him, to want two ice creams in one day. I was jealous of *my own son!* It makes me sick to my stomach to realize I did to him what my mother did to me. *More than anything else, I don't want to be like my mother.*

Lillian Rubin has spent her life trying to separate from her mother. She says:

> I've spent my life in a love-hate ambivalence with my mother, trying to reach her at the same time that I moved as far away as I could. There were periods, sometimes years, when I actually believed I had left her behind—that I had rooted her out of my inner life, that I had completed my lifetime project of disidentifying with her—only to find her popping back again at some unexpected moment.[2]

In her memoir, *Remind Me Who I Am, Again,* author and journalist Linda Grant writes:

> I was a feminist, I was a Marxist, I wanted the world turned upside down, but principally I wanted more than anything else not to be like my mother.[3]

Like Lillian Rubin, Linda Grant's mother constantly changed history. Both mothers refused to admit things that transpired earlier. This is very unsettling because it is both infuriating and undermining. "It was not a household which valued the truth . . . So I knew I came from a long line of accomplished liars." And like Lillian's mother, Linda's mother was angry and unloving. She says: "I was not a happy child."

> And this may have been because motherhood—at least of young children—was not one of my mother's talents. I grew up assuming that my mother did not particularly like children . . . I do not think she would have chosen motherhood if there had been any realistic alternative. She would, I think, have preferred to maintain her position as beloved child bride to a man fourteen years older than her.[4]

Nevertheless, the mother's terminal phase of life can offer an opportunity for reparation and growth. Understanding the childhood feelings that emerge during caregiving can transform the terminal period from simply a time of emotional pain and loss for a daughter into a final opportunity for her to develop as an autonomous woman.

When Linda Grant became the caregiver to her mother, who suffered from multi-infarct dementia, she looked at her mother in a new way:

> I see then that the mother in whose eyes I was a failed daughter is gone. That I am never going to win the great argument with her about the kind of daughter she expects me to be for my adversary has left the field.[5]

How does a daughter who never had an intimate relationship with her mother deal with taking care of her mother when she suffers from dementia? When asked if she loves her mother, she responds:

> But do I love my mother? I will collude in the public con-
> vention that children love their parents and none more re-
> servedly than when they are cast into the role of "carer."
> But at least it's true that I care what happens to her.[6]

Ellen Gulden, the daughter who goes home to care for her dying mother in Anna Quindlen's novel *One True Thing,* only discovered who her mother was and what she meant to her during the months she cared for her. While Lillian Rubin and Linda Grant spent their lives trying to disidentify with their mothers and did so long after their mothers died, Ellen was finally able to identify with her mother after a lifetime of disidentifying with her because of her wish to identify with her idealized father instead. The months spent caring for her mother allowed Ellen to pare her father down to size and begin to appreciate the enormity of her mother's positive impact on her.[7]

Unlike the fictional Ellen Gulden, writer Louise DeSalvo was not able to work through her feelings about her mother before she died. In her memoir, *Vertigo,* DeSalvo describes her memory of the years she had with her mother while her father was off in the war and her sister was not yet born. When the men left, life took on an antic, festive, tribal quality.

> The women who were left behind . . . threw open all the
> doors to their apartments and children began to clatter up
> and down the five flights of stairs at all hours of the

day and night. Women and children wandered from one apartment to another without ceremony or invitation.[8]

DeSalvo says that although the women *said* they missed their men, they were far happier when the men were gone. Her idyllic time with her mother ends with her father's return. Her father did not represent pleasures separate from her mother. On the contrary, she experienced her father as an interloper and spoiler.

> Nighttime story hours were shortened or curtailed altogether. Snacks were forbidden. Mothers hushed their voices and hushed us, to listen with deference and awe to whatever the men had to say.[9]

Even after her mother dies, Louise still experiences her father as intruding on the intimacy she had with her mother. A few weeks after her mother's death, he gives Louise an envelope her mother left for her. But he makes it clear that he read it first.

Her sister, Jill, is another intruder—not so much in her life as in her suicidal death.

> In the years that have intervened since my sister's death, my mother's pain is clearly visible, ever present. She stops enjoying my children. She stops enjoying our family gatherings. She stops enjoying everything. Her mouth is permanently drawn downward into a frown. When we take family pictures, she forces a smile. She pushes herself, each day, through her routine, through her life. She isn't with us, though. She's with Jill.[10]

Louise suffered from depression her entire life—her mother's death is the *fourth* time she experienced losing her mother—when her father returned from the war; when Jill was born and completed the separation of "us wartime children from our mothers"; when Jill hung herself; and finally when her mother died. By the time her mother dies, she is so full of pent-up rage and depression that she cannot mourn her. Instead, she tries to hold on to her by identifying with her in the way that Freud described in *Mourning and Melancholia.* Freud says: "The ego wishes to incorporate this (lost) object into itself."[11] Louise says:

> I think my life is beginning to resemble my mother's. I don't go out of the house except to do my exercise walking or unless I have to. I stop seeing my friends. I cancel speaking engagements. I'm afraid to go anywhere, afraid . . . to live my mother's life, and in this way, I'm trying to keep her alive.[12]

Louise was not able to work through her anger at her mother at the end of her mother's life. Five years after her death, however, she asks: "How can a woman mother when she hasn't herself been mothered?" That is substantially different from what she told a friend the day her mother died: "I never had a mother, and now she's dead."

Louise's anger at her father and sister as the interlopers who took her mother away from her covers a deeper and even more painful reality—her mother's inability to mother. Louise's grandmother died in the influenza epidemic of 1918, when Louise's mother was two. Her grandfather farmed his daughter out to relatives and friends and finally married a woman who chided her stepdaughter with "You're not my blood." Louise's mother was depressed before Louise was born—she looks depressed in her honeymoon pictures.

WARDING OFF
A NEEDY MOTHER

Susan is a fifty-one-year-old marriage counselor. She and her husband and two daughters live in a large home in Brooklyn. When I arrived for our interview, she greeted me warmly and asked if I'd like a cup of tea. We talked in a sun-filled room with several couches with lots of pillows to lean on. She's a comfortable, low-keyed woman who seems very clear about who she is.

Susan grew up in California. Her mother, Sophie, had a chronic spinal condition as a result of whiplash from an auto accident when Susan was a young girl. During Susan's teen years, her mother suffered more and more neck pain. She had two surgeries, but the damage was never completely repaired. She was functional, but in pain, and then she got arthritis and it became more and more debilitating.

Susan says her mother's constant emotional pain preceded her physical problems. Sophie's mother died when she was eight years old. To compensate for her own wish to be mothered, she wanted to be "an ever-present, always-there mother"—the mother she never had: "But," Susan says, "I took care of her a lot emotionally. I was like *her mother.* She depended on me for that kind of closeness." Susan says her father was a kind and caring man, but he was not emotionally or physically there for her mother: "Her needs were enormous and my father's gratification was in his work." Susan's father was a physician who worked evenings and weekends. Susan's brother was not available to help Susan manage her mother's dependence on her either. They were never close as children because of their age difference—he went off to college when Susan was eight. Her father's absence and her brother's distance left Susan alone with her mother's neediness. She felt that she was drowning in it. Susan says:

> I needed to separate myself—to say, "I'm going to have my own life." Coming back to care for her made things complicated.

The pull to take care of her mother emerged again when her father died. Her parents moved from their house to a condo and her father started to slow down at work so that they could spend more time together. About a year later, he was taken to the hospital in severe pain three months after bypass surgery. After he died they realized that he had an infection in his tooth that had traveled to his aorta. Although this would have been terrible for any woman, for Susan's mother it was an even more severe trauma.

Susan says that before Sophie got cancer, she visited her mother twice a year and her mother visited her twice a year. Susan needed to keep her distance, across the country, so that she would not be overwhelmed by her mother's neediness.

> I wasn't angry at the end going to take care of her, but I was angry earlier, after my father died, when I felt she wanted me to take care of her. When I thought of her coming to live with us, I was frightened.

She says it was hard to leave her children and care for her mother when she was dying. But she explains:

> I wanted to do it. I wanted to comfort her. It felt like the right thing to do. At the end, when I was there, I was bathing her and emptying her bedpans. It's tough doing that for your mother. Seeing her so weak and deteriorated was painful. There was a piece of it that felt good, yes it was hard, but I could do it anyway.

Taking care of her mother emotionally was something that Susan was used to. The role reversal went all the way back to her childhood. Then she rebelled against it; she moved far away from her mother. She saw an ocean of neediness and turned and ran. However, when her mother was diagnosed with terminal cancer, there was something specifically wrong with her. And she was dying—it would not go on forever as Susan feared.

> When she got sick, I didn't felt guilty because then there was something definite wrong and I wanted to take care of her. At the end I was going every three weeks. It was after my father died and she was alone and lonely for twenty years that I didn't want to take care of her.

Once she was diagnosed with cancer, her mother's neediness had limits and Susan felt safe enough to respond. Indeed, she got in touch with her wish to take care of her mother.

A FATHER-DAUGHTER ROMANCE

While the child's relationship with the mother is originally a twosome and the triangular element (that is, mother, child and father) emerges later, the child's relationship with the father is a triangle from the beginning. For the girl, typically, her father is a deliciously intriguing person who is the first person outside the mother-daughter orbit. However, this was not the case for Louise DeSalvo, who experienced her father as disrupting the mother-child dyad. Fathers usually play an important role in helping daughters differentiate from their mothers and realize that being feminine doesn't mean being Mommy—there are ways of being feminine and yet different from Mommy. On the other hand, if the father demeans his wife to his daughter, the daughter grows up with ambivalent feelings about being a woman and a wife/mother.

Later, fathers become the center of a little girl's romantic fantasy and her competition with her mother. Optimally, the father is able to lovingly support and appreciate his daughter's emerging femininity, while making it clear that he has a special relationship to Mommy that is separate from her. With that kind of father, the girl is able to grow up feeling attractive and comfortable with herself—loving her father, but looking for another man to satisfy her adult needs. If her father is too gratifying (that is, makes her feel that he prefers her to her mother), it might be hard for the daughter to find any other man who can match him in her eyes—a recipe for disappointment.

Erica is an example of a daughter whose romance with her father made it difficult for her to invest her emotional energy in either of her two husbands.

Erica recounts:

My father took us on an ocean liner to Europe. They had a movie theater on the ship and I went with my sister to see *North by Northwest*. The man at the door asked how old I was and I said: "I'm eleven and a half." He said I couldn't go in. You had to be twelve. I was very upset and ran to get my father. He came down with me and said to the man: "It's true that my daughter is eleven and a half, but she is more mature than most twelve-and-a-half-year-olds. Please let her in."

Erica cries when she tells the story. Her father just died and no one will ever protect her, stand up for her and think she is as special as he did. I feel envious of her loss in a way. "My father wrote me a poem every night. He'd come into my room at bedtime and read me a book or talk to me about my day and then he would write a poem on my blackboard. It was this special thing between us." Erica felt her father was intensely interested in her—her friends, her day at school and her songs. Because my relationship with my father was so different, I was always surprised when Erica would tell me she invited her friends to dinner with her parents. I wondered to myself: Why would your parents want to spend the evening with your friends? It was unthinkable for me that my parents would want to spend time with my friends. My parents never remembered my friends' names; they never talked to them; they never asked me to tell them about my friends. I was shocked that she felt her father was interested in her friends and was delighted to see them and learn about them. She invited her friends to visit with her father in order to please him.

When her father had congestive heart failure and grew weary of his failing body, Erica sang to him, cooked for him, brought friends to cheer him and took him to a psychiatrist for antidepressants. Erica felt angry with her mother for not taking good enough care of him—for not loving him as much as she did. She also began to understand why there was a lack of intimacy in both her marriages. She remained "Daddy's girl." Erica feels that no other man took care of her the way her father did and no other man can make her feel as special as her father. In contrast to Erica's father, my father made it abundantly clear that his special relationship was with my mother.

MY FATHER had congestive heart failure for about fifteen years before he died in 1996. During that time he would go to the emergency room several times a year because his lungs filled with fluid, and a few times he had pneumonia. Several times when he thought he was dying he said to me or my sister or brother: "Take care of Mom." The first few times he said this to me I felt furious, although I didn't show it. I wanted to yell at him: "All you ever think about is taking care of her. You're my father and you're dying. Why can't you say: 'I love you' or 'Be good to yourself' or 'I'm proud of you'? Why is your last communication the same as it has always been: 'You're not on my mind, I'm only interested in your mother'?"

At seventy my father was the star part-time salesman at Nat Sherman, the tobacco shop. He loved to regale us with tales of selling fancy humidors to wealthy cigar smokers. He worked at Nat Sherman's until he had his first heart attack in the store—they were not interested in having him return. He had gotten the job there after retiring from Bayside Oil, where he was a salesman and owned one-seventh of the company (two trucks). He was at Bayside for about ten years before he retired. For over thirty years before he went to Bayside he worked for the Hunter Coal Company on Flatbush Avenue in Brooklyn. But when people stopped heating their homes with coal the company went out of business. It was just before my parents' twenty-fifth anniversary trip to Fort Lauderdale, Florida. My father, as usual, wanted to protect my mother; he did not want to upset her before the trip. He told my sixteen-year-old sister what happened, but he asked her to keep the secret from my mother. He did not seem to understand that he was asking my sister to bear the burden instead of my mother.

My father was a short, bald, paunchy Jewish man, and my mother constantly ignored his wishes, disregarded his opinions and insisted that he be subjugated to her mother and her sister Gus. Most of the time he silently acceded. There are a few memorable occasions, however, when he stood up to my mother or my aunt and seemed heroic in my eyes.

When Eisenhower ran against Stevenson, my father was probably the only Jew in Brooklyn who voted for Ike. When my mother's family gathered one Sunday night at Aunt Mitzi's house, Gus (knowing that my father was the Lone Ranger voting for Ike) went around the room asking people for whom they were voting. When she got to my father, he said, "I'm voting for Ike," and she started screaming at him. When my parents returned home that night in 1952, I remember my mother was not speaking to my father because he had gotten up and walked out when Gus started screaming at him. He had done the unspeakable—he stood up to Aunt Gus.

When my sister wanted to move out of the family apartment and share an apartment with a friend in Greenwich Village, my father stood up to my mother and supported my sister's moving on. And when I wanted to go to the University of California at Berkeley rather than Brooklyn College, my father once again stood up to my mother. But there were not many other times; most of the time my father sacrificed all of us (himself, my brother, my sister and me) to please my mother.

For many years I was enraged at my father for not protecting us (or himself) from my mother and Aunt Gus. He was a collaborator and the three of us were the Allies. Our war continued during the Vietnam years when I was in the antiwar movement, which began at Berkeley during my college years. My father supported the war with all his heart. Perhaps you heard us yelling at each other?

When I returned home from college I got an apartment in Greenwich Village (like my sister before me) and began psychoanalysis and graduate school. I remained rather distant from my father for many years—interspersed with conversations that increased the distance. For example, I wrote this poem about my father thirty years ago—before I met my husband.

MY FATHER LOVES ME

Yes, there is no doubt that my father loves me.
He worries when I sound down on the phone,
And tries to pick me up with kind words.
"Mrs. Sweeney is 68 and she met a man on a cruise . . .
If Mrs. Sweeney can get a guy so can you . . ."
I note the kindness in his voice
I know the reason why I'm crying isn't because I think he's
    mean.
I know my father loves me.
That's why he's telling me this.
After all, Mrs. Sweeney is 68. Mrs. Sweeney is a widow.
Mrs. Sweeney is fat and ugly. But, of course . . .
Mrs. Sweeney is rich. But men aren't interested in that any-
    more.
I didn't yell at my father.
I didn't even tell my mother to yell at my father.
I didn't want to be mean to my father because
He didn't mean to be mean.
I know my father loves me.

I felt angry that my father was so distant. I felt he never
saw me. He had no idea how pained I was about not being
able to find a man I could love. My father could not deal with
emotions; he used aphorisms instead, for example, "better
dead than red." I wanted him to understand what mattered
to me; I wanted him to see me as a woman and understand
my yearnings. But he never did.

In the last year of my father's life, he began to stand up to my mother and I began to understand why he could not do it when my sister, brother and I needed him to. My father's father died when he was a little boy—maybe four or five. I remember a picture of my father at about that age dressed in a cowboy outfit. He always said that was from the time they lived out west in Arizona or New Mexico briefly before my grandfather died of tuberculosis at thirty-two. My grandmother, a beautiful woman of thirty, was left with two little boys, my father and his younger brother, Bob. My father never talked much about his childhood except to say that his mother married a nasty man who owned a grocery store and she used to steal from the till because he was so cheap. She never loved her second husband; she married him out of desperation when she returned to New York.

But at the end of his life, my father was able to share more about his early life. He told my sister that when his mother returned to New York as a widow, she almost put the boys in an orphanage. Instead she decided to marry a man she didn't love who could support her and her children. But she was not a warm or loving woman, and I guess my father grew up wanting to win her love. Instead, he married my mother and spent his life trying to get *her* to love him. He was willing to do whatever she wanted to win her love. He gave money to her family; he took insults from her sister Gus; he accepted her unwillingness to have anything to do with his mother; he stood by mutely when she screamed at us endlessly and slapped me across the face until her hand hurt.

By the end of his life, I could forgive him. A few months before he died, my parents went to Florida and my father slipped in the bathroom. He went to a rehabilitation hospital in Miami for six weeks, but they told us they could not keep him there longer. He needed to be transferred to a nursing home or a rehabilitation facility that worked with people on a long-term basis. My brother went to Florida and brought my parents back to New York. My sister and I met them at the rehabilitation hospital in Coney Island when the three of them arrived from the airport at midnight by ambulance.

My brother was distraught from the experience of dealing with my father's incontinence and my mother's neediness on the plane. So he left immediately and went on vacation. My sister and I took over arranging things for my father's care and consoling my mother. He was in that facility for about a month or so before he died of congestive heart disease. I visited him twice weekly before going to teach my classes at Brooklyn College. He was in a rehabilitation hospital, but he did not want to do any of the exercises. He did not want to get out of bed. When I visited him, my mother was often there. But she didn't hold his hand or stroke him. I don't think my mother has ever been able to offer comfort to anyone—I have never experienced or witnessed it. I wanted to comfort him. I was able to feel that he was grateful for the times I fed him in his hospital bed and put cream on his dried and irritated arms and legs. He was grateful that I held his hand and kissed his face. It makes me cry as I write this, but it feels good because it's loving and not angry.

DAUGHTERS CARING for mothers frequently reexperience anxieties about merging and losing themselves in their mothers' neediness—particularly the daughter who feels her mother was always needy. Susan worked hard to stay separate from her mother and resented her neediness. But when her mother was diagnosed with terminal cancer and Susan knew it would not go on forever, she was able to take care of her mother without being overwhelmed. On the other hand, daughters who devalued their mothers, like the fictional Ellen Gulden, often find caregiving an opportunity to connect with their mothers for the first time. Sometimes a woman, like Maria in Chapter 6, finds caring for her mother an opportunity to have the intimacy with her that she never was afforded as a child.

While issues of identification and separation are central to the mother-daughter relationship, oedipal issues are often at the heart of the father-daughter relationship. I wanted to be more special to my father than my mother was; I wanted him to reject her because she was not comforting and turn to me. I was competing with my mother for my father's love. That's why it felt so painful to me to hear my dying father say: "Take care of your mother" rather than "Take care of yourself."

Taking care of the parent of the opposite sex revives old passions and conflicts, just as parenting does. In order to neither be seductive nor turn away from your child's sexuality in a way that is experienced as rejecting, a parent has to accept his/her own attraction and desire for the child of the opposite sex and then find an appropriate way to express it. Similarly, when daughters care for their fathers they regress and early feelings for the father emerge. This is what happened to Erica. While other daughters might find the feelings too threatening and turn away, Erica was quite comfortable with her feelings about her father, perhaps too comfortable. But if you can accept the feelings and find an appropriate way to express them, the caregiver experience can feel healing and life-affirming.

Chapter Eight

SONS

Whosoever knows the latitudes of his mother's body, whosoever has taken her into his arms and immersed her baptismally in the first-floor tub, lifting one of her alabaster legs and then the other over its lip . . . whosoever has kissed his mother on the part that separates the lobes of her white hair and has cooed her name while soaping underneath the breast where he was once fed . . . who has pushed her discarded bra and oversized panties (scattered on the tile floor behind him) to one side, who has lost footing on these panties, panties once dotted with blood of children unconceived, his siblings unconceived . . . to lift up his stick figure mother and to bathe her ass, where a sweet and infantile shit sometimes collects . . . whosoever slips his mother's panties up her legs and checks the dainty hairless passage into her vulva one more time, because he can't resist the opportunity here for knowledge . . . he shall never die.[1]

WHY DOES NOVELIST RICK MOODY follow these descriptions of son-mother intimacy and sexual connection and transgression with the phrase "he shall never die"? It seems to be the opposite of what we might expect—that a son would be struck dead for such inappropriateness.

Hex Raitliffe, the "hero" of *Purple America,* returns home to care for his paralyzed, incontinent, almost mute mother who is suffering from a degenerative neurological disease. In the one night in which the novel takes place, beginning with bathing his mother, we experience Hex's unsuccessful attempt to blot out his angry, sexualized relationship with his mother. Hex utters all the unspeakable thoughts and emotions that most men repress.

Moody describes Hex caring for his mother: "Her son tries to anticipate her needs, to preempt her need for words, to eliminate a language based on need, and thus to eliminate language." Hex feels so merged with his mother that words are unnecessary. Would being fully separate from his mother be the equivalent of dying?

Achieving manhood involves separating from the mother— the man must renounce his bond to his mother and enter into a new and independent social status recognized as different, even opposite, from hers. Thus the boy's development is, in many ways, more difficult than the girl's. The little boy has to differentiate himself and his maleness from his mother's femaleness even though she is the person on whom he is totally dependent. This process of differentiation or disidentification is a central part of a boy's inner life.

As a result of this essential need for the boy to disidentify with his mother, the movement away from the mother begins earlier in boys than girls. He has to extricate himself from the mother-infant oneness, but wants to know that his mother is still available to him if he needs her. The danger of merging with the mother is the boy's greatest anxiety; if he surrenders to his wish to return to that delicious infantile oneness with her, he fears both the loss of his identity as a separate self and the loss of his masculinity. If the boy's struggle to disengage from the mother is overly stressful, he may surrender and not develop a sense of masculinity and separateness or he may overcompensate and develop a macho veneer.

Adult sons are often more comfortable having physical contact with their fathers rather than their elderly mothers. Many sons, unlike Hex Raitliffe, are loathe to care for mothers because of the need to disidentify from the mother and defend against the wish to merge with her, as well as the need to disavow any sexual feelings toward her.

Although most adult children who are caregivers of elderly parents are female, the gender of the parent determines, in part, whether the daughter or son is the primary caregiver. While daughters are more likely to be caregivers than sons in general, when sons are primary caregivers, it is more likely to be for their fathers than their mothers.

A man who is the primary caregiver for his mother probably will have to confront challenges to his earliest and most fundamental concept of himself. Brought up to emphasize cognitive over emotional aspects of experience, socialized to provide and protect, he is now required to nurture. He is required to do "women's work." While all of the men in this chapter were nurturing as caregivers, Jonathan is the only one who feels comfortable talking about the emotional aspects of the experience. Repressing their emotional reactions seems to be part of the disidentification process. That is what makes Rick Moody's book so shocking—nothing is repressed.

Some sons become caregivers to their parents at a point in their life cycle when they are naturally more expressive and nurturing. As men approach middle-age they tend to integrate more of a range of feminine and masculine characteristics. They are less threatened by the feminine dimensions of their selves and feel less of a need to prove their masculinity.[2] Still, for a son to take responsibility for the physical care of his mother is fraught with the potential of having to deal with conflicts about his mother that, for some men, have remained unresolved since childhood. We can see, then, that for many sons being the primary caregiver to a mother is fraught with psychological danger.

CARING FOR MOM WHEN DAD WAS NEVER IN THE PICTURE

Ken is a fifty-four-year-old teacher. Gruff and heavyset, he was surprisingly willing to talk about his painful relationship with his mother, who had died fifteen years before. He told me he never talked to any of his friends about this, but he was eager to talk to me. Ken's parents were quite well-to-do. His father was a successful doctor and the family was financially comfortable until his parents separated when he was ten years old. Ken says his father was an alcoholic and "out of the picture" even when he was little. When I asked him about what he meant, it became clear that his father was never *in the picture with his mother*. His father was present, but there was no positive connection between his father and mother, so Ken felt that he had to take care of his mother. When his father got drunk, he hit her. Ken says: "I was left

222 ◆ DOING THE RIGHT THING

trying to protect my mother from my father. My brother was too young. I felt I had to take care of her."

When his parents separated, Ken's protectiveness toward his mother intensified. Ken explained that he could not separate from his mother. When he was a boy, he got so hysterical when she wasn't around that he was sent to a child psychiatrist. The treatment enabled him to separate enough to go off to college. But after college he came back to live with his mother for many years until he got an apartment in the same building.

Ken's younger brother, who was brought up by a nanny, moved to California when he went to college and never came back. In contrast, Ken says he always felt responsible for his mother. He recounts:

> She went through periods of tremendous anxiety. She couldn't cope. She'd be fine for a week or a month, but she was nervous and paranoid. She might have been manic-depressive. She was in therapy and on psychotropic drugs. It was extraordinarily difficult to care for her, but I didn't resent it. She'd call me twelve times a day.

Ken says he didn't resent it, but he was depressed and became alcoholic:

> The alcohol helped me deal with all the stress. I was dependent on it. But I only missed one day of work in all those years. It didn't hurt my functioning. I would drink a half a bottle of whiskey every night. I'd start drinking at 5:30 or 6 and drink until 10 and go to bed.

Ken had no relationships. He said he could not relate to women; he calls it "arrested development." His friends believed he would never get married, but they did not understand that his relationship with his mother was at the heart of the problem. All he did was work, drink and care for his mother. His mother would call him hysterically and he ran to her. Ken says meeting his wife was the turning point in his life: "I told her what was going on and she understood. I moved in with her right away." What his wife, Pam, "understood" was that Ken could not separate from his mother. He had a difficult time telling his mother that he was getting married. He said: "I think she was relieved and happy but also threatened."

Ken's mother killed herself three months after he got married. As insightful as he is, Ken attributes his mother's overdose to her feeling that he was happy and she "had no reason to hang in there anymore." He does not seem to want to know that she might have killed herself because she felt she had lost him and couldn't live without him. When he found her dead, he said, it was devastating, but a relief. He was finally free to have a life. But it was not so easy for him to have a separate life after all those years of being so intimately connected to his mother.

> I wasn't sure I would be able to do it. I drank a lot. But five years ago the doctor said I can't drink anymore because I have a heart condition. I had to do it and so I did it. I stopped.

Had Ken's father been more available, Ken's separation problem with his mother might have been less extreme. The father plays a decisive role in the boy's struggle to disengage from the mother and be able to experience emotional and physical pleasures away from her. The father is a masculine alternative to the feminine mother, an other-than-mother figure. The boy can strive to be like his father and acquire his power. However, Ken's father did not help him disengage from his mother. On the contrary, his father put Ken in the position of having to take care of his mother (because of his absence) and protect her (because of his abuse). That prevented Ken from being able to separate from his mother and develop relationships with other women. The result was isolation, depression and alcoholism. The symbiosis between them was so extreme that when Ken was finally able to separate, with the help of his wife-to-be, his mother killed herself.

SHOWING APPRECIATION
FOR A MOTHER WHO "WAS THERE"

Bob is an attractive sixty-five-year-old African-American man. He is married with two grown children, a son who is an attorney and a daughter who is a college professor. He is a retired technical training manager for a phone company. He has been retired for eleven years.

Bob's mother is eighty-eight and comes to the senior center five days a week. Physically, she is in good shape, but she has Alzheimer's disease. She was diagnosed eighteen years ago and his father cared for her at home for two years before he died.

Bob is the third of four brothers. After his father died, one of his brothers offered to oversee the mother's finances and have his son and his wife move into Bob's mother's house. They would care for her and live there rent-free. But the son and daughter-in-law could not cope with caring for an elderly woman with Alzheimer's. They moved out and Bob started getting calls from two of his brothers and the nephew who had lived with his mother telling him that the brother who was overseeing the finances was "not doing right." After the young couple moved out, Bob's brother was locking his mother in the house for the day and spending her pension money. He took all the knobs off the stove so she wouldn't start a fire, but she wasn't being fed, clothed or cleaned properly. Finally, Bob's other brothers and nephew asked Bob to take care of her. Bob says he had a conference with his wife and children and told them it would be a long haul—three to ten years. They all agreed to do it. Bob says the adjustment was not easy:

> It was hard for me to make the transition from child to parent. This is a child that doesn't get older, but younger. I had to wash her, clean her and take her to the bathroom. At the beginning she was conscious of being bare. It wasn't easy.

But Bob says it's a daily routine now.

> Monday to Friday my wife and I get her up, take her to the bathroom, get her washed, give her breakfast and get her out of the house between 9 and 10:30 a.m. My wife is a registered nurse and has experience with Alzheimer's patients. We take her to the center every day.

Bob's mother can't talk anymore. And he misses being able to go to events or travel. However, Bob says that it is hard to get respite care:

Our biggest problem is we have no time for ourselves. Getting child-care is easy, but getting care for someone with Alzheimer's is not easy. People don't understand elderly people. It's harder to be with them. You can't play with them like you can play with a child. It's not fun. You can't just get a teenager from down the street.

I asked Bob if he ever thought about putting his mother in a nursing home. He said:

I don't trust nursing homes. I've never seen an effective one. The staff in nursing homes is not compassionate. People have bedsores or don't eat. They put down the food and expect you to eat it, and if you don't they take the plate away. If I paid $40,000 a year we would find compassionate people, but I can't.

But the more we talked, the more it became clear that money is not the reason Bob does not put his mother in a nursing home. Although he doesn't say it, it seems obvious that caring for his mother had a great deal to do with his decision to retire so early. Bob wants to take care of his mother. His wife is willing to have his mother live with them and she does a lot of caregiving. But Bob says:

It's *my* mother, so if my wife has a meeting to go to or wants to go to the movies with her sisters, she goes and I stay with my mother. I cook, I clean, I wash clothes—we both do it.

I wondered why this sixty-five-year-old man is willing to bathe his mother and take her to the bathroom. Why is he willing to give up the benefits of being financially comfortable and fancy-free? Bob explained why he feels that he can't do enough for his mother.

I wasn't the best child. I was in trouble. I used to steal. I'd stay out late at night. I hung out with a bad crowd—a gang called the Casanovas. The thing that changed my life at sixteen was that the guys I was with robbed a store on a Saturday night and I was with them. On Monday, they all got arrested. Some got probation and some went to jail because they had prior records. I was afraid to go home. I told my parents I was there but I didn't do anything and they decided I should live at my aunt's house for a while. To this day I don't know why the police never came for me.

I was shocked. I could not imagine this warm, mild-mannered man with such an easy laugh being a juvenile delinquent! Clearly something important changed in him as a result of such a close call with the law. I could see that he was grateful to his parents for protecting him when he was so frightened. He told me that all of his neighborhood friends were either in prison or had been murdered. But was that enough to explain having his mute mother with Alzheimer's living with him for almost twenty years? Then Bob told me another story about his parents that made me understand how deeply he loves his mother and wants to care for her.

When I was eighteen I developed tuberculosis and I was in the hospital for two and a half years. It was like leprosy, no one came to visit me. People were too frightened. Only my mother and father came to visit me. Every day they came—they were always there. When I fell down they always picked me up.

Bob describes his parents as his "shield" and his "crutch." He said he could always lean on them. In return, he says:

I never borrowed money from them. I only gave to them and I could never give them enough. To this day I feel like I haven't given her enough.

At that point Bob asked me: "Did you meet her?" Since I had not, he took me out to the main room to meet his mother. "Isn't she pretty?" he asked. "Yes," I said, "she *is* a pretty woman." His mother was a petite woman dressed in a lovely outfit and her white hair was coiffed attractively. She smiled at me blankly, not having any idea who I was.

CARING FOR AN ADORED FATHER

When I entered the church looking for Tom's office, I was aware of a certain formality in the surroundings. I wasn't sure the interview would be useful because I imagined the minister I was about to meet would be a formal man who had the "right" feelings about his parents and would speak in aphorisms. Can a minister talk about ambivalence, I wondered to myself as I reached the door of his office? When I stepped into Tom's office, all those questions fell away. His office was messy with books and jazz CDs. He welcomed me warmly and seemed eager to talk. As we sat down to talk, Tom told me that yesterday would have been his father's ninety-ninth birthday.

Tom's caregiving began several years ago when his father, who had been caring for his mother, who had Alzheimer's, didn't answer the phone. Tom called the police and they broke into the apartment and took his father to the hospital. He had had a stroke. Tom rushed to New York to pick up his mother and bring her to his house in Connecticut. His mother lived with Tom, his wife and two children for a little while, but he and his wife felt caring for someone with Alzheimer's was overwhelming for the family, so they put her in a nursing home.

When his father got out of the hospital, Tom brought him to live with his family. After being with them for a short time his father developed a blood clot in his leg and needed an operation. When he got out of the hospital, Tom got him a room in the same nursing home as his mother. Tom says:

> He was never independent after that. I saw him every day for four years until he died. I can be pretty oblivious to un-pleasantness. I felt it was primal. If I hadn't done it, I would have missed out on one of life's essential duties. I felt it was my duty, but also my privilege. There's war, there's famine, there's pestilence and there's parents.

Tom's mom died two years before his father. He said she didn't know where she was or what was going on around her most of the time.

With my mother, the caregiving experience wasn't good. When she was out of it, it didn't bother her. I could walk past her room and feel like she didn't know the difference. When she knew how diminished she was, it was hard to bear.

But Tom had a different kind of experience caring for his father. Tom's father had been a professional football player—quite a famous one it seems. He played for eight years in the NFL, from 1926 to 1933. Tom felt very proud of his father and enjoyed how outgoing he was and how much people liked him: "Everybody loved my father. The nurses would bring him takeout food. They'd ask for his autograph." Tom told me that as a kid he adored his father. His favorite song was "Oh My Papa."

Tom idealizes his father. His eyes twinkle when he tells me about him. When he walked down the street, people knew him and they would call out, "Hi, Rob." When his father retired from football, he was a buyer for a large electric company. His father had contracts to buy millions of dollars of merchandise. As a result, he got very generous Christmas gifts from the companies from which he bought goods. There was cognac and scotch; hams and turkey; flowers and plants; cigars and cigarettes; wines and cheeses. Every New Year's Eve Tom's parents gave a party and all their neighbors and friends would come and indulge in the luxuries provided by his father. He says:

My father used to make a hell of a good drink before dinner and we would get blasted together when I was in college and graduate school. When he was at the nursing home, we'd sit and watch ball games and drink beer and it reminded me of those old days and it made me smile.

Tom felt his father was appreciative and it felt good to him. He told me life was chaotic, but it was convenient. The nursing home is down the block from the church. His wife would say, "Why do you have to go over there today?" But Tom wanted to see his father every day. The day his father died, he and his wife were going shopping at the mall and Tom wanted to stop and see him. His wife didn't want to and then finally said, "I'll wait in the car. Hurry up." His father died that night. I wondered if Tom felt guilty or upset that he wasn't there when his father died. He said, "I didn't feel I had to be there the moment he died. A lot of people put a lot of pressure on themselves. I didn't."

Suddenly, I realized why Tom, who seemed so unlike any expectation I had of a minister, *was* a minister—probably a wonderful minister. He said, "You have to forgive yourself. You can't worry about what you *can't do.*" Tom accepts his own limitations. He forgives himself. He explains:

When this all started, I had a new job, two young children and my father and mother were both here needing care. There were three things tugging at me. I felt if I think about what I *can't* do, I will be overwhelmed, so I have to think about what I *can* do and not worry about the rest of it.

Tom's worldview is one of acceptance. For example, he talked about getting annoyed at his father.

My annoyance could be brought up with a phrase like: "Whatcha been doin'?" Which meant "Where have you been?"

Tom said he sees other people lose their temper with their parents and he is very calm and professional. But with his father it was different. He wasn't calm and professional—he was often annoyed or angry. For example, his father would say: "You said you'd be back in a minute and it's been five minutes."

My biggest fear was my last encounter with him would be angry. But then again you're giving them dignity by being pissed off at them. It's real. There were stresses.

So Tom got angry and felt guilty about it: "Sometimes I was disappointed in myself that I couldn't get over that initial childhood reaction of being pissed off." But then he forgave himself. He told himself it was better to be emotional and attached and treat his father like a person who affected him, not an old man who was not worth getting angry at. He is humorously self-effacing, but underneath it is self-forgiveness:

I can get into arguments all by myself. I can just go to the meat counter and argue about whether to get the pork chops or the chicken.

Tom's acceptance of himself applies to other people as well, like his brother, John. Tom's wife got angry when John visited. "Why didn't your brother offer to pay for half of the Chinese dinner?" "Why doesn't your brother get up and clear the dishes?" Tom says his brother was used to having his meals served to him and being viewed as an authority. Tom says he and John live in different worlds.

> We were on different sides of the Vietnam War and we had to come to an accommodation with each other about who we were. Sometimes his attitude would amaze me. He would come up to visit my parents and he would read the newspaper and not talk.

Tom is shocked that his brother described his childhood as being like the Harry Chapin song about a father who's always busy and the son keeps asking: "When are you coming home, Dad?" Then the son grows up and never has time for his father. Tom did not experience his father as unavailable and distant, but John did.

Tom explained that he and John grew up in different worlds. John was born in 1940 and Tom was born in 1947. His mother told him childrearing philosophy was turned on its head between 1940 and 1947. John was brought up on the advice of Dr. Spock: Feed the baby every four hours. Disregard the screaming. Don't comfort the baby or you will encourage him to keep crying in hopes of getting picked up. Let the baby cry until he gives up hope of comfort. The baby must learn to tolerate frustration and to wait for the next feeding.

As our interview was coming to an end, Tom showed me an article he wrote about his father after he died. Tom collected all the newspaper clippings and pictures of his father's football career and interviewed some of his surviving teammates. Tom said his father didn't talk much about his "glory days," but after his death Tom set out to get a full picture of his father's football career. In the article, Tom quotes a woman who wrote him a sympathy note when his father died. She was a cheerleader for a team his father coached in the years before World War II. She wrote: "He was an idol to the players. They were awed that they had this great star as their coach." He was an idol to his son Tom as well.

When I read Tom's article about his father, I thought about my writing about my parents. Both of us used writing as a way of pulling together fragments and seeing our parents as whole people. But I was struck by the difference between what I am writing about my parents and what Tom wrote. Tom's article was about the facts of his father's football career—the number of games, the number of passes, the number of yards. It was about his father. My writing is not simply about my mother and father, but my *relationship with my mother and father.* Our ways of putting our parents to rest seem not only to reflect the difference in our feelings about them, but also our genders. He wrote about the facts and I wrote about the feelings.

TRYING TO FORGIVE
AN ALCOHOLIC FATHER

Remember Jonathan from Chapter 4? Jonathan is an only child caring for his eighty-two-year-old mother, who has bipolar disorder. Before his father died a year and a half ago, Jonathan was the primary caregiver for his father as well because his mother was unable to care for him. In order to do that, Jonathan had to confront his intense anger at his father for being sadistic to his mentally ill mother; for being critical and judgmental of him; for not taking care of him when he was a child and his mother was in mental hospitals; and for being an alcoholic.

Unlike Tom, who idealized his father and embraced his father's lifestyle and values, Jonathan feels contemptuous of his father's values and has spent his life trying not to be like him. He says:

> My parents were very much like the Cleavers—they wanted everything to be perfect. They wanted to wear the right clothes, have their kids go to the right school, belong to the right club, hang around with the right people and make the right connections. They were very much from that sort of Republican girl-boy network kind of a mold.

Jonathan sees his father as trying to please his grandfather. Jonathan's contempt is even more visceral when he talks about his grandfather, who he calls "Mr. Assimilation." Jonathan recalls:

> My father's father came from Switzerland. He was Roman Catholic, but when he came here he became Presbyterian. My grandfather was very successful in business and made a lot of money and he wanted to assimilate. He wanted my father to be the perfect American boy—go to Taft, go to a good college, work in New York, wear a dark suit and a white shirt and do everything by the book.

Jonathan feels that his father's need to please his grandfather led him to give up his own dreams and live the life his grandfather prescribed for him.

My father wanted to be a landscape architect, so he had to repress his interests to follow the paint-by-the-numbers lifestyle that his father demanded of him. My impression is that my father was totally programmed.

In contrast to his father, Jonathan gave up a job he never enjoyed and began studying social work at forty-eight. While that was a rebellion of sorts for Jonathan, it is not surprising that he chose a career of helping families in trouble considering his family's history.

Jonathan's father was severely wounded in World War II and spent two years in the hospital. He was one of the first patients in the United States to receive extensive reconstructive surgeries over a two-year period. He was listed for amputation, but his arm was saved. However, as a result, his physical skills were compromised. When Jonathan was a child, his father couldn't play ball. A lot of the physical things that a father wants to do with his son, he was not able to do. He had huge grafts taken out of his abdominal area, and his arm was deformed. Jonathan says that it also affected his father's body image.

In addition, Jonathan's father came home from the war with post-traumatic stress syndrome—he had flashbacks and nightmares.

I can remember waking up as a kid, on a number of occasions, where he was awake, his eyes were open, he was cradled in my mother's arms, screaming, "Medic, medic, I'm hit!" crying. Tears were streaming. I remember as a small child walking into the room, just thinking, "All right, he's not dreaming because his eyes are open." I had no explanation; I had no frame of reference for it. My mother would just say, "Your father's okay. Don't worry." She would hold him the moment that he was hit by the mortar shell.

After the war, Jonathan's father became an alcoholic. He never drank during the week, but was drunk all weekend. Jonathan says that when his father drank, he was cruel and verbally abusive.

One night we were in the kitchen and my father was drunk. He said to my mother: [imitating his father in a loud, raspy voice] "Go ahead, goddamn it, tell him. Tell him you're a Jew!" You know, I wanted to kill my father. Thank God there wasn't a gun in the house.

Jonathan felt enraged at his father's cruelty toward his mother—particularly the way he used Jonathan against her.

I would say to my father, you know I'm really concerned about Mom. He would then get her behind closed doors and say, "See, see what's happening? Your son knows it. Your son can see what's happening. Would you pull yourself together? Look what you're doing. Look what you're doing to this family." That was the way my father was—he thought depression was just a bad attitude. Just get rid of the bad attitude and get on with life.

Jonathan says that his father was extremely judgmental when he was a child. He used the same tone and language with Jonathan that he did with his mother. Jonathan recalls learning in psychology class that you are supposed to talk to the person about their behavior. You don't want to erode the person's self-esteem. You want to help the person develop a mindset that will increase their self-esteem. But Jonathan says his father was the opposite. What he did was the antithesis of focusing on the behavior rather than the person. He describes his fear of his father.

> I remember I would get very poor grades in math. I would come home from school with my report card. And I would sit on the back porch. I would sit on the milk box, petrified. I'd sit there till it was dark, it'd be after dark, and I'd hear my parents in the kitchen: "Where is he? Do you think he's okay?" My mother would start making phone calls. Then, all of a sudden, someone might come to the window and see me, or I'd get up and walk in through the door. I'd show him the report card. It was never: "You know you're doing well in the other subjects." He'd say: "You're never gonna get into college."

Jonathan was alone with his father during the times his mother was hospitalized. He was drunk a lot of the time. In 1973, when Jonathan was a senior in college, his mother tried to kill herself with alcohol and pills—it was her second or third suicide attempt. His mother was hospitalized again and his father was drinking excessively. Jonathan says his father had been drunk, disruptive and verbally abusive on Christmas Eve. When Jonathan came downstairs on Christmas morning he confronted his father. He says:

> I said, "Okay, I'm having you committed." My grandfather's sitting there in his three-piece suit, just looking

shocked, speechless, looking at us. His eyes were going back and forth like he was watching a tennis match. I said, "You're out of control. I'm going back to school. My mother is in an institution. You're no good to anybody, including yourself, right now. I can't leave you like this because you're crazy, so I'm calling the state hospital." He said, "No, no, no. You can't do that, put down the phone, put down the phone. I'll go to Alcoholics Anonymous."

Jonathan called Alcoholics Anonymous and they sent somebody over that afternoon to meet with his father. They gave him a mentor and he got into the program. Jonathan went to Alcoholics Anonymous meetings with his father for three weeks during semester break. When he returned to college after his Christmas break, his father started drinking again and stopped going to meetings. Jonathan pleaded with him to go back to AA, but his father cried on the phone and told him: "You don't understand what it's like to be married to your mother and have to go through this."

Jonathan got teary at this point and told me that at the time he was in his last semester of college and they offered him an opportunity to graduate with honors, but he had to take comprehensive tests. He turned down the opportunity because he was so emotionally drained from dealing with his mother's suicide attempts and his father's alcoholism. He felt he could not sit for the tests.

I called my father back and I said, "All right, here's the deal: I don't need you anymore. I'm going to have a college degree. It's paid for. You can't stop payment on your check now. I'm going to get a job. If you ever want to see me

again you both have to stop drinking. That's my deal."
They both stopped drinking. That was 1974.

Ironically, Jonathan's father was diagnosed with cancer just
as Jonathan was leaving his job and preparing to enter the
social work program. He became afraid that once again he
was going to have to sacrifice school because of his father.
All his old fear and anger surfaced once again:

> I was so upset because I was taking a psychology course
> and I had to take a week off. I had to have somebody else
> get notes for me. I was afraid of failing. My fears turned
> out to be unfounded. But I guess I had a lot of pent-up
> emotions about that.

Jonathan feels his father's derogatory attitude toward him
has had tremendous ramifications in his life. After college,
Jonathan went to Harvard at night to take pre–social work
classes. He recalls:

> There were no pressures, nobody knew about it. I was pay-
> ing for it. I got straight A's. But I still, to this day, question my
> ability. I'm petrified of getting a B. To me, a B is a failure. I
> put this huge pressure on myself to be a straight-A student.

But Jonathan did not go to social work school then. He took
a job doing something that didn't interest him. He put his
dreams aside—just like his father did. But now, he says:

> I'm making up for what I missed. I have a feeling that on the
> one hand, I'm very lucky to have this second chance at the

career I always wanted. On the other hand, because I have this second chance, I cannot screw up. I've got to be perfect.

Jonathan still struggles with trying to please the father he has internalized, an abusive and sadistic father—his alcoholic father. Jonathan has to be perfect and get all As to please that internal father. Jonathan also struggles with his identification with that father. He says he's gotten more control over it in recent years, but he is afraid of it reemerging under the pressure of caring for his mother.

> I could be very volatile at times. I could be very cruel to people. I modeled my father's behavior. If I was depressed, if I was not feeling good about myself, which was a lot of the time, I could be really nasty to people. It was like Abbott and Costello, you know how Abbott was supposed to be his friend but he always used to turn on him and be nasty? I could never watch Abbott and Costello because it used to remind me of myself.

Jonathan's father turned over all his financial assets to Jonathan a year before he died. That vote of confidence from his father meant a great deal to him.

> The fact that it was really a clear-cut decision that this was what he wanted to do and that it would be a relief to him to do it meant a lot. This wonderful change has occurred and it really changed the way that the family has dealt with one another. It gave him a feeling of relief and it gave me a feeling of relief because I wanted to have a little bit more control in order to help them.

Jonathan feels that he was able to work through his feelings about his father before he died. They talked a lot about what had gone on between them. When his father was dying Jonathan told me:

> I really squared things with my father. The air is clear. It has really improved. Do I love him? I always have. But I love him unconditionally now. And I forgive and I forget and I think he forgives and we have a wonderful relationship now.

While Jonathan was able to work through his angry feelings toward his father before he died, he still struggles with his identification with him—particularly in relation to his mother. His father blamed his mother for not being able to function. He made her feel that she was being selfish or spoiled when she was overcome by depression. Jonathan struggles with trying to accept that his mother is not capable of taking care of herself. He reverts back to trying to get her to make decisions and getting frustrated and angry at her when she cannot, but then he reminds himself that she is sick—and he isn't a little boy.

CARING FOR a mother brings up any unresolved conflicts about physical intimacy and separation a man might have. The fictional Hex Raitliffe struggled with his sexualized relationship to his mother. Like Hex, Ken struggled with his inability to separate from his mother. It made him depressed, alcoholic and unable to have a relationship with a woman until he was in his forties and met his wife. Bob, on the other hand, has cared for his mother for many years, but his relationship with his mother does not seem to be fraught with sexual or separation conflicts. He loves his mother, but he does not seem to be psychologically entangled with her. He and his wife of more than thirty years care for his mother together, and he seems to feel very warm and loving toward her.

Caring for a father can offer a man an opportunity to be close to his father in a way that he was not able to as a child. It can also evoke a different set of psychological conflicts than caring for a mother. For Tom, caring for his father was an opportunity to spend time with an adored father. Tom did not have to overcome intense anger at him or the wish to not be like him. Jonathan, on the other hand, had to work through intense anger at his father and confront his strong wish to disidentify with him.

Caregiving that goes beyond financial control or mowing the lawn can be more stressful for men than women because men are less likely to have friends or family with whom they discuss emotional issues. Ken never talked to his friends or his brother about what he was going through with his mother. His wife was the first person with whom he ever discussed it. For many men, the experience of being the primary caregiver is the first time they have thought about how they *feel* about their parents. For those who allow themselves to know what they are feeling, it can be a rich, if painful, experience.

HOW CAN I HANDLE THIS BETTER?

C. WRIGHT MILLS WROTE: "Perhaps the most fruitful distinction with which the sociological imagination works is between the personal *troubles* of the milieu and the public *issues* of social structure."[1] "Troubles" occur within the character of the individual and his immediate relations with others. "Issues" transcend the individual and his inner life—they have to do with the organization of many milieus to form the larger structure of social and historical life.

Doing the Right Thing is about the connection between individual troubles and a major contemporary social issue. The social issue is the increase in the number of elderly people (13 percent of Americans). The troubles are the experiences of those of us who have to care for our elderly parents in a society in which there has not been provision for their care—only their longevity.

Taking care of an elderly parent is not like taking care of a child. Instead of fostering healthy growth and autonomy, you are witnessing slow or, in some cases, rapid deterioration. Instead of watching a child's world open up and expand, you are watching your parent's world contract. In contrast to a child's having his or her life ahead of them, an elderly parent is facing death ahead.

However, one important reason that parent care is like parenting is that it revives powerful elements of the original parent-child relationship. Caregiving reactivates daughters' feelings of dependency, needing to be understood and yearning for appreciation and approval. Caregiving evokes the vestiges of a daughter's oldest fantasies about her mother—it makes her regress. It awakens childhood feelings you didn't know you had or you thought you had left behind a long time ago.

You remain a child no matter how old you are because that old lady is *your mother.* For example, when my friend Alexandra visits her mother and she says, "Oh, I'm so happy to see you, I'm so glad you came," Alexandra doesn't feel like an adult. She told me, "I smile at her and give her a kiss on the cheek, but what I *feel* is: 'You never said that to me in all these years. You had to have lots of mini-strokes in order to express any positive feelings to me.'" After many years of psychoanalysis, finally getting her mother's appreciation still throws her back into the pool of rage she thought she left behind many years ago.

Most of the caregivers I interviewed did not experience taking care of their elderly parents as giving "payment" for services rendered. Indeed, many felt their parents had given them insufficient love and/or protection, neglected or abused them or entrusted their care to surrogates such as nannies. Only one caregiver, Bob, felt that he was paying his mother back for saving him from a life of crime and for the comfort she provided when he was hospitalized for tuberculosis as an adolescent. Why are people who feel they were not loved or adequately taken care of by their parent willing to take care of that parent? For many there's a deep yearning for appreciation. It's a final attempt to be recognized as a "good daughter" or "good son"—worthy of the love never given.

Author and social worker Vivian Greenberg calls the caregiving stage "the last dance." The last dance is unique because it symbolizes the end. Parents and children who have bungled earlier stages have a harder time with the last one—they are used to two solos. The last dance can be the final heart-wrenching disappointment or it can be a coming together in love and forgiveness.[2]

The child who is the primary caregiver is often *not* the child who was closest to the parent or has the best relationship with the parent. Often, the caregiver is the child who is still trying to work out an unresolved conflict about the parent. The caregiving period then becomes the stage for repeating old conflicts—or, as we have seen in some cases, an opportunity for finally working through those conflicts. Sometimes it is worked through with the parent, but, unfortunately and perhaps more often, it is worked through by the caregiver alone.

So how do we find meaning and comfort in this phase of our relationship with our parents? My philosophy is that there are no one-size-fits-all answers. But there is a way of thinking about the difficulties that caregiving brings that can help us find our own custom-made answers. Caregiving forces us to think about our relationship with our parents—the past one and the present one. It makes us examine our values and priorities; what makes us feel good about ourselves and what makes us angry; what makes us feel guilty and what makes us feel peaceful. In order to use the opportunity to know our selves and our parents better, we have to be willing to listen to our feelings even when they are ambivalent and even if we wish they were different.

We don't necessarily have to act on our feelings, because feelings and actions are separate. But knowing what we feel helps us decide whether we *want* to act. For example, you may want to have your mother live with your family, but you have to ask yourself some questions: How will I feel if I act on that wish (heroic, good about myself, angry and resentful)? What level of care will she need? Am I willing to provide that? What will I have to give up (time alone with my husband, friends, children or grandchildren or work responsibilities)? What will my husband and children have to give up (privacy, vacations and dinner out)? How will I feel about my mother as a result of her moving in?

After considering the answers to these questions and discussing them with family members, you may decide you do want to act on your wish to have your mother live with you. But you may realize you need to make provisions for private time, monetary compensation or out-of-home care. However, you may also decide not to act on that wish because you have a host of other feelings that militate against doing it. If you accept that you wish you could make the offer, it can soothe you to know that you want to help your mother. However, if you decide the negative consequences are too great, allowing yourself to feel both sides of the ambivalence can help you think of another option that will allow you to be as generous as you can without feeling stuck in an intolerable situation. You will be able to give yourself permission to look for an alternative that gets your mother the care she needs and also makes you feel comfortable. As one of my patients, who has a very difficult time tolerating her ambivalent feelings, said to herself: "Don't try to erase the ambivalence, weigh the valences."

Of course, no one likes to face the fact that a parent is dying. No matter how old you are, and how difficult your relationship with your parent might have been, facing their death means confronting that you don't have parents and you are soon to be the older generation. You will eventually have to come to grips with the issue of your own old age. But the last years of a parent's life can be a time when we can choose to work out conflicts that have plagued us for most of our lives. And perhaps, if we are lucky, we may develop a richer, deeper relationship with our parent before he or she dies and be able to remember our parent with love, warmth and acceptance.

In order to maximize the chances of making that happen, we have to first accept the fact that ambivalence is a natural and normal part of caregiving—for the caregiver as well as the elderly parent. The caregiver has to make personal sacrifices and struggle with anger and guilt, while the elderly parent has to give up their autonomy and allow themselves to depend on their children. With all the best intentions, caregiving is fraught with emotional conflict.

You also have to hold on to the reality that when you face your parent's ocean of neediness, the best you can do is bring a cup. Setting limits helps protect you from drowning as well as from feeling that you have to turn and run away. In that way it protects your parent as well because it *enables you* to help. It prevents you from getting stuck in a cycle of anger and guilt.

It is also important to pay attention to anger and guilt as signals that you have to understand, but not necessarily act upon. If you try to ignore those feelings and push on, they get worse. You may not express your anger directly, but forget to call your mother or meet her at the doctor. Or, worse yet, you may notice that you're getting headaches more often, yelling at your children or drinking excessively. If you are feeling angry or guilty, find someone to talk to about it. Angry feelings are a signal that you need to rethink your limits and/or that old, unresolved feelings are reemerging. Maybe you can talk to a friend or join a support group. If you find that you can't control your anger and/or guilt, it may help to find a therapist who can help you sort out the old feelings that are interfering in your caregiving.

It is important to remember that you have obligations and responsibilities in addition to any caregiving you take on. Those obligations cannot be abandoned for caregiving. You have obligations to your spouse, children, employer—and to yourself. Obligations have to be weighed against one another. An important meeting with your boss may trump your usual visit to your mother. Going to the mall to shop for college with your daughter may trump having your father to dinner.

You have to find a balance between being humane and not being self-destructive—your own personal way of bringing a cup. Not everyone will agree about what that involves. Some of your friends may feel it's terrible to put a parent in a nursing home, while others may feel that it is self-destructive to do anything else. Finding what you can comfortably give is something you have to find out for yourself because no one else can tell you what will make you feel good, angry or guilty.

However, I think there are some questions that you can ask yourself to help sort out whether your caregiving is destructive for you, your family or your parent.

1. Are you getting depressed, having anxiety attacks or getting physically ill from it?
2. If you are married or in a relationship, is that relationship suffering as a result of your caregiving? If you are not in a relationship, is the caregiving preventing you from having one?
3. Are your children being neglected (because of your absence or distraction) or abused (because you're in a bad temper) as a result of your caregiving?
4. Are you following a cultural script that is consistent with your own values? Or are you doing what you think other people expect or what you think you "should" do?
5. Does caring for your parent make you feel good or bad about yourself?
6. Are you giving something positive to your parent that he or she could not otherwise get? Or are you making a big sacrifice to do something that is only marginally important?
7. Are there options you are not considering out of hand or because of things you promised years ago that are no longer feasible?

As caregivers, we have to make peace with the reality that our parent is going to die. Despite our efforts, death is inevitable. All we can offer is comfort and support. We are limited in what we are able to do.

However, some of you also have to make peace with the fact that you have parents who will not accept your comfort and support—or will not acknowledge it. A difficult parent may have always been difficult and as he or she gets older those problems do not disappear. A father who was an alcoholic at forty may still be an alcoholic at eighty; a mother who had a personality disorder when she was thirty will most likely still have it at eighty-five. Illnesses and losses of later life can make a dependent personality more dependent; a controlling parent who feels out of control, more controlling; a self-centered parent even more focused on his or her own needs.[3]

On the other hand, your elderly parent's personality may have become difficult as a result of the death of a spouse or sibling, or a chronic illness. The latter case is easier to handle because there is hope that your parent can change with the help of medication, counseling or mourning. In the former case, however, when your parent has had these personality problems your whole life, you are most likely to repeat an interaction with him or her that was developed in childhood. For those of you who are struggling to care for a difficult parent, it is even more imperative to set limits that you and your family can live with and to pay attention to the warning signs that you are entangled in an old dynamic.

When our parents are old and soon going to die, we yearn for them to account for their lives. What do they feel good about and what do they wish they had done differently? Why did they treat us the way they did? What was going on in their lives that made them treat us that way? Some people are very lucky and get to have that life accounting with their parents. The bad news is that most of us are not so lucky. We have to do it ourselves or with the help of a therapist. The good news is that we can find peace. Peace may come from the satisfaction that you can have those conversations with your own children before your life is ending, even if you could not have them with your parents. Peace may come from understanding the historical and intergenerational context of our parents' way of treating us. Peace may come from knowing and accepting that you are separate.

NOTES

Introduction

1. Victoria Secunda, *When You and Your Mother Can't Be Friends* (New York: Delta, 1992), p. 4.

2. Arlie Russell Hochschild, "The Sociology of Feeling and Emotion: Selected Possibilities," in M. Millman and R. M. Kanter, eds., *Another Voice: Feminist Perspectives on Social Life and Social Science* (Garden City, NY: Anchor Press/Doubleday, 1975), pp. 280–307.

3. U.S. Department of Health and Human Services. 1999. *Health, United States, 1999: Health and Aging Chartbook*. DDHS Publication number (PHS)99-1232-1: 58. Also see Emily K. Abel, *Who Cares for the Elderly? Public Policy and the Experiences of Adult Daughters* (Philadelphia: Temple University Press, 1991).

4. Deborah M. Merrill, *Caring for Elderly Parents: Juggling Work, Family, and Caregiving in Middle and Working Class Families* (Westport, CT: Auburn House, 1997), p. 2.

5. Erik H. Erikson, *Identity, Youth and Crisis* (New York: W. W. Norton and Company, 1968).

6. In his famous essay about the life cycle, Erik Erickson posited eight stages in the life cycle—each one characterized by a central inner conflict. For example, the seventh stage, middle adulthood, spans the middle twenties to the fifties. Erikson says the central conflict is gen-

erativity vs. stagnation. Generativity is contributing to the welfare of future generations. It can take the form of having and raising children or it can take other forms—for example, teaching, writing or social activism. Stagnation, on the other hand, is being self-absorbed and not concerned about your legacy to future generations. Erikson's eighth and final stage is late adulthood, which begins in our sixties and lasts to old age. During this final stage of life the central conflict is ego integrity vs. despair. We either come to terms with our life and our impending death or we experience despair. Some people come to grips with their choices and mistakes and develop a sense of wholeness that Erikson calls "ego integrity." Other people become preoccupied with their failures and the losses that are part of aging—loss of friends, relatives and spouse. They feel despair.

7. Anna Quindlen, *One True Thing* (New York: Dell, 1994), p. 304.
8. http://www.thefamilycaregiver.org
9. U.S. Department of Health and Human Services. *Health, United States, 1999.*
10. Gail Sheehy, *The Silent Passage* (New York: Pocket Books, 1998), p. 247.
11. Abel, *Who Cares for the Elderly?*
12. http://www.thefamilycaregiver.org
13. Merrill, *Caring for Elderly Parents,* p. 3.
14. Psychoanalysts such as Margaret Mahler have talked about the process of "separation-individuation" in the first three years of life. "Individuation" is the process of developing psychological autonomy—perception, cognition and reality testing. "Separation" is the process of differentiating from the mother and developing boundaries. Margaret S. Mahler, Fred Pine, and Anni Bergman, *The Psychological Birth of the Human Infant* (New York: Basic Books, 1975).
15. The term "good-enough mother" was coined by D. W. Winnicott. Winnicott said the good-enough mother provides a "facilitating environment" for the infant to go through the maturational process. In contrast to Winnicott, I am using the term "mother" to refer to the person who is the primary caregiver—it could be a grandmother or a nanny or an aunt or a father. Similarly, I am referring to the mother as "she," because the primary caregiver is usually a woman, but it could be a man as well. D. W. Winnicott, *The Family and Individual Development* (London: Tavistock Publications, 1965).
16. Peter Blos, *On Adolescence* (New York: Free Press, 1962), p. 12.

17. Psychoanalyst Melanie Klein argued that all infants go through a stage in which they "split" the mother into an ideal, need-satisfying mother and a depriving, frustrating mother. Klein contended that adequate mothering allows the child to eventually put the two images of the mother together and be ambivalent. However, if the mothering is not adequate, the child needs to maintain the ideal image of the mother in order to keep it separate from the "bad mother." Hanna Segal, *Introduction to the Work of Melanie Klein* (New York: Basic Books, 1964).

18. Secunda, *When You and Your Mother Can't Be Friends,* p. 15.

19. Ibid.

Chapter One. Setting Limits

1. The term "attachment," which has been used loosely in caregiving literature, is based on John Bowlby's life-span attachment theory. Life-span attachment theory is based on the concept of infant attachment—the emotional bond between the infant and the mother or main caretaker. It is important to remember that attachment is an internal state within the individual. To the extent that the child finds comfort and security in the mother, the child forms a secure attachment and an internal feeling of the attachment figure as responsive and supportive. Although secondary attachments develop throughout life, the primary attachment colors the later ones. The primary attachment is maintained over distance and time; it is carried inside you. If it was a secure attachment, the adult continues to experience the feelings of comfort and security by symbolically representing the absent parent through memories, shared values and interests. John Bowlby, *Separation: Anxiety and Anger. Attachment and Loss Volume II* (New York: Basic Books, 1973).

2. Psychoanalysts call this phenomenon "transference."

3. Judith Viorst, *Necessary Losses* (New York: Simon and Schuster, 1986), p. 22.

4. Anne Wilson Schaef, *Co-Dependence: Misunderstood-Mistreated* (San Francisco: Harper, 1986).

5. Melody Beattie, *Codependent No More* (Center City, MN: Hazelden Information and Education Services, 1987).

6. Wendy Lustbader, *Counting on Kindness* (New York: Free Press, 1991).

7. Vivian E. Greenberg, *Respecting Your Limits When Caring for Aging Parents* (San Francisco: Jossey-Bass Publishers, 1989).

Chapter Two. Getting Angry and Getting Over It

1. Harriet Lerner, *The Dance of Anger: A Woman's Guide to Changing the Patterns of Intimate Relationships* (New York: HarperCollins, 1997), p. 112.
2. "Working through" is a process that is central in psychoanalysis and psychoanalytic psychotherapy. In psychoanalytic work the early experience is reexperienced with the analyst in a process called "transference." It's in the current experience with the analyst that the patient comes to understand and digest the early experience or trauma. The process of working through allows the patient to distinguish past and present and eventually move on without unknowingly repeating the early trauma over and over.
3. Lustbader, *Counting on Kindness*.

Chapter Three. Feeling Guilty and Forgiving Yourself

1. This desperate plea for help was posted on the discussion forum of Caregiver.com.

Chapter Four. Spouses

1. Roberta Satow, ed., *Gender and Social Life* (Needham Heights, MA: Allyn & Bacon. 2000).
2. Ibid.
3. Ibid.
4. Susan Forward. *Emotional Blackmail: When the People in Your Life Use Fear, Obligation and Guilt to Manipulate You* (New York: HarperCollins, 1997).

Chapter Five. Siblings

1. Stephen P. Bank and Michael D. Kahn, *The Sibling Bond* (New York: Basic Books, 1982), p. 16.
2. Jane Mersky Leder, *Brothers and Sisters: How They Shape Our Lives* (New York: Ballantine Books, 1991), p. 2.
3. Merrill, *Caring for Elderly Parents,* p. 101.
4. Julie Robison, Phyllis Moen, and Donna Dempster-McClain, "Women's Caregiving: Changing Profiles and Pathways," in *Journal of Gerontology: Social Sciences,* Vol. 50B, No. 6 (1995), S372.
5. Lenard W. Kaye and Jeffrey S. Applegate, *Men as Caregivers to the Elderly: Understanding and Aiding Unrecognized Family Support* (Lexington, MA: Lexington Books, 1990), p. 7.

6. Abel, *Who Cares for the Elderly?* p. 5.

7. Greenberg, *Respecting Your Limits When Caring for Aging Parents.*

8. Ada C. Mui, "Caring for Frail Elderly Parents: A Comparison of Adult Sons and Daughters," in *The Gerontologist,* Vol. 35, No. 1 (1995), pp. 86–93.

9. Mary Ann Parris Stephens, Melissa M. Franks, and Audie A. Atienza, "Where Two Roles Intersect: Spillover Between Parent Care and Employment," in *Psychology and Aging,* Vol. 12, No. 1 (1997), p. 35.

10. Abel, *Who Cares for the Elderly?* p. 107.

11. Sarah Fenstermaker Berk, "Women's Unpaid Labor: Home and Community," in *Women Working: Theories and Facts in Perspective,* 2nd ed., edited by Ann Helton Stromberg and Shirley Harkess (Mountain View, CA: Mayfield Publishing, 1988).

12. Karen L. Fingerman, *Aging Mothers and Their Adult Daughters: A Study in Mixed Emotions* (New York: Springer Publishing Company, 2001), p. xiii.

13. Ibid.

14. Mario Tonti, "Relationships Among Adult Siblings Who Care for Their Aged Parents," in *Siblings in Therapy: Life Span and Clinical Issues,* edited by Michael D. Kahn and Karen Gail Lewis (New York: W. W. Norton and Company, 1988), pp. 417–34.

15. Bank and Kahn, *The Sibling Bond.*

16. Ibid., p. 109.

17. Sarah H. Matthews, "Gender and the Division of Filial Responsibility Between Lone Sisters and Their Brothers," *In Journal of Gerontology: Social Sciences,* Vol. 50B, No. 5 (1995), S312–S320.

Chapter Six. Cultural Scripts for Caregivers

1. Ann Willard, "Cultural Scripts for Mothering," in *Mapping the Moral Domain: A Contribution of Women's Thinking to Psychological Theory and Education,* edited by Carol Gilligan (Cambridge, MA: Harvard University Press, 1988), pp. 225–43.

2. Although caregiving is predominantly women's work, care of the elderly is largely absent from the feminist agenda in the United States. Feminist scholars lavish attention on motherhood, but they continue to slight other forms of unpaid work, such as caring for elderly parents. Both forms of private domestic labors are undervalued because they are outside the economy. See Berk, "Women's Unpaid Labor: Home and Community."

3. Abel, *Who Cares for the Elderly?* p. 4.
4. Charlotte Ikels, "The Process of Caregiver Selection," in *Growing Old in America: New Perspectives on Old Age,"* edited by Beth B. Hess and Elizabeth Markson (New Brunswick, NJ: Transaction Books, 1985), pp. 136–50.
5. U.S. Bureau of the Census, 2000. "Relationship by Household Type (Including Living Alone) for the Population 65 Years and Over," Summary File 2, PCT 21.
6. Christine L. Himes, Dennis P. Hogan and David J. Eggebeen, "Living Arrangements of Minority Elders," in *Journal of Gerontology: Social Sciences,* Vol. 51B, No. 1 (1996), pp. 542–48.
7. Lisa Groger, Pamela S. Mayberry, Jane K. Straker and Shahla Hehdizadeh, "African-American Elders' Long-Term Care Preferences and Choices." Final Report, Award #90-AR-2034 (Washington, DC: Administration of Aging, Department of Health and Human Services, August 1997).
8. Carole Cox and Abraham Monk, "Strain Among Caregivers: Comparing the Experiences of African-American and Hispanic Caregivers of Alzheimer's Relatives," *International Journal of Aging and Human Development,* Vol. 43, No. 2 (1996), pp. 93–105.

Chapter Seven. Daughters

1. Linda Grant, *Remind Me Who I Am, Again* (London: Granta Books, 1998), p. 38.
2. Lillian B. Rubin, *Tangled Lives: Daughters, Mothers, and the Crucible of Aging* (Boston: Beacon Press, 2000), p. 49.
3. Grant, *Remind Me Who I Am, Again,* p. 46.
4. Ibid., p. 78.
5. Ibid., p. 166.
6. Ibid., p. 265.
7. Quindlen, *One True Thing,* p. 53.
8. Louise DeSalvo, *Vertigo: A Memoir* (New York: Dutton, 1996).
9. Ibid., p. 56.
10. Ibid., p. 245.
11. Sigmund Freud, "Mourning and Melancholia," in John Rickman, ed., *A General Selection from the Works of Sigmund Freud* (New York: Doubleday, 1957), p. 131.
12. DeSalvo, *Vertigo,* p. 252.

Chapter Eight. Sons

1. Rick Moody, *Purple America* (Boston: Little, Brown and Company, 1997), pp. 3–4.
2. Kaye and Applegate, *Men as Caregivers to the Elderly*, p. 14.

Conclusion. How Can I Handle This Better?

1. Mills, C. Wright, *The Sociological Imagination* (New York: Grove Press, 1959), p. 8.
2. Vivian E. Greenberg, *Children of a Certain Age: Adults and Their Aging Children* (New York: Lexington Books, 1994), p. 163.
3. Grace Lebow and Barbara Kane with Irwin Lebow, *Coping with Your Difficult Older Parent: A Guide for Stressed-Out Children* (New York: Avon Books, 1999), p. 8.

BIBLIOGRAPHY

Abel, Emily K. *Who Cares for the Elderly? Public Policy and the Experiences of Adult Daughters* (Philadelphia: Temple University Press, 1991).

Aranda, Maria P., and Bob G. Knight. "The Influence of Ethnicity and Culture on the Caregiver Stress and Coping Process: A Sociocultural Review and Analysis." *The Gerontologist* 37, 3 (1997): 342–54.

Bank, Stephen, P., and Michael D. Kahn, *The Sibling Bond* (New York: Basic Books, 1982).

Beattie, Melody. *Codependent No More* (Center City, MN: Hazelden Information and Education Services, 1987).

Berk, Sarah Fenstermaker. "Women's Unpaid Labor: Home and Community." In *Women Working: Theories and Facts in Perspective,* 2nd ed. Edited by Ann Helton Stromberg and Shirley Harkess (Mountain View, CA: Mayfield Publishing, 1988).

Berman, Claire. *Caring for Yourself While Caring for Your Aging Parents* (New York: Henry Holt and Company, 1996).

Biegel, David E., Esther Sales, and Richard Schulz. *Family Caregiving in Chronic Illness: Alzheimer's Disease, Cancer, Heart Disease, Mental Illness and Stroke* (Newbury Park, CA: Sage Publications, 1991).

Blos, Peter. *On Adolescence* (New York: Free Press, 1962).

Bowlby, John. *Separation: Anxiety and Anger. Attachment and Loss Volume II* (New York: Basic Books, 1973).

Cox, Carole, and Abraham Monk. "Strain Among Caregivers: Comparing the Experiences of African-American and Hispanic Caregivers of Alzheimer's Relatives." *International Journal of Aging and Human Development,* Vol. 43, (2) (1996), pp. 93–105.

DeSalvo, Louise. *Vertigo: A Memoir* (New York: Dutton, 1996).

Erikson, Erik H. *Identity, Youth and Crisis* (New York: W. W. Norton and Company, 1968).

Fingerman, Karen L. *Aging Mothers and Their Adult Daughters: A Study in Mixed Emotions* (New York: Springer Publishing Company, 2001).

Forward, Susan. *Emotional Blackmail: When the People in Your Life Use Fear, Obligation and Guilt to Manipulate You* (New York: HarperCollins, 1997).

Freud, Sigmund. "Mourning and Melancholia." In John Rickman, ed., *A General Selection from the Works of Sigmund Freud* (New York: Doubleday, 1957).

Grant, Linda. *Remind Me Who I Am, Again* (London: Granta Books, 1998).

Greenberg, Vivan E. *Children of a Certain Age: Adults and Their Aging Children* (Lexington, MA: Lexington Books, 1994).

———. *Respecting Your Limits When Caring for Aging Parents* (San Francisco: Jossey-Bass Publishers, 1989).

Groger, Lisa, Pamela S. Mayberry, Jane K. Straker and Shahla Hehdizadeh. "African-American Elders' Long-Term Care Preferences and Choices." Final Report, Award #90-AR-2034 (Washington, DC: Administration of Aging, Department of Health and Human Services, August 1997).

Groger, Lisa, and Pamela S. Mayberry. "Caring Too Much? Cultural Lag in African-Americans' Perceptions of Filial Responsibilities." In *Journal of Cross-Cultural Gerontology* 16 (2001), pp. 21–39.

Himes, Christine L., Dennis P. Hogan and David J. Eggebeen, "Living Arrangements of Minority Elders." In *Journal of Gerontology: Social Sciences,* Vol. 51B, No. 1 (1996), pp. 542–48.

Hochschild, Arlie Russell. "The Sociology of Feeling and Emotion: Selected Possiblities." In M. Millman and R. M. Kanter, eds., *Another Voice: Feminist Perspectives on Social Life and Social Science* (Garden City, NY: Anchor Press/Doubleday, 1975).

Ikels, Charlotte. "The Process of Caregiver Selection." In *Growing Old in America: New Perspectives on Old Age,"* ed. Beth B. Hess and Elizabeth Markson (New Brunswick, NJ: Transaction Books, 1985).

Kaye, Lenard W., and Jeffrey S. Applegate, *Men as Caregivers to the Elderly: Understanding and Aiding Unrecognized Family Support* (Lexington, MA: Lexington Books, 1990).

Lebow, Grace, and Barbara Kane with Irwin Lebow. *Coping with Your Difficult Older Parent: A Guide for Stressed-Out Children* (New York: Avon Books, 1999).

Leder, Jane Mersky. *Brothers and Sisters: How They Shape Our Lives* (New York: Ballantine Books, 1991).

Lerner, Harriet. *The Dance of Anger: A Woman's Guide to Changing the Patterns of Intimate Relationships* (New York: HarperCollins, 1997).

Lustbader, Wendy. *Counting on Kindness* (New York: Free Press, 1991).

Mahler, Margaret S., Fred Pine and Anni Bergman. *The Psychological Birth of the Human Infant* (New York: Basic Books, 1975).

Matthews, Sarah H. "Gender and the Division of Filial Responsibility Between Lone Sisters and Their Brothers." In *Journal of Gerontology: Social Sciences.* Vol. 50B, No. 5 (1995), S312–S320.

Merrill, Deborah M. *Caring for Elderly Parents: Juggling Work, Family, and Caregiving in Middle and Working Class Families* (Westport, CT: Auburn House, 1997).

Mills, C. Wright. *The Sociological Imagination* (New York: Grove Press, 1959).

Mui, Ada C. "Caring for Frail Elderly Parents: A Comparison of Adult Sons and Daughters." In *The Gerontologist,* Vol. 35, No. 1 (1995), pp. 86–93.

Moody, Rick. *Purple America* (Boston: Little, Brown and Company, 1997).

Olson, Laura Katz, ed. *Caring for the Elderly in a Multicultural Society* (Lanham, MD: Rowman and Littlefield Publishers, 2001).

Pyke, Karen. "The Micropolitics of Care in Relationships between Aging Parents and Adult Children: Individualism, Collectivism, and Power." In *Journal of Marriage and the Family,* 61, 3 (1999), pp. 661–72.

Quindlen, Anna. *One True Thing* (New York: Dell, 1994).

Robison, Julie, Phyllis Moen and Donna Dempster-McClain. "Women's Caregiving: Changing Profiles and Pathways." In *Journal of Gerontology: Social Sciences,* Vol. 50B, No. 6 (1995), S372.

Rubin, Lillian B. *Tangled Lives: Daugters, Mothers, and the Crucible of Aging* (Boston: Beacon Press, 2000).

Satow, Roberta, ed. *Gender and Social Life* (Needham Heights, MA: Allyn & Bacon, 2000).

Schaef, Anne Wilson. *Co-Dependence: Misunderstood-Mistreated* (San Francisco: Harper, 1986).

Secunda, Victoria. *When You and Your Mother Can't Be Friends* (New York: Delta, 1992).

Segal, Hanna. *Introduction to the Work of Melanie Klein.* (New York: Basic Books, 1964).

Seltzer, Marsha Mailick, and Lydia Wailing Li. "The Dynamics of Caregiving: Transitions During a Three-Year Prospective Study." *The Gerontologist,* Vol. 40, No. 2 (2000), 165–78.

Sheehy, Gail. *The Silent Passage* (New York: Pocket Books, 1998).

Stephens, Mary Ann Parris, Melissa M. Franks and Audie A. Atienza. "Where Two Roles Intersect: Spillover Between Parent Care and Employment." In *Psychology and Aging,* Vol. 12, No. 1 (1997), p. 35.

Tonti, Mario. "Relationships Among Adult Siblings Who Care for Their Aged Parents." In *Siblings in Therapy: Life Span and Clinical Issues,* ed. Michael D. Kahn and Karen Gail Lewis (New York: W. W. Norton and Company, 1988), pp. 417–34.

U.S. Bureau of the Census. "Relationship by Household Type (Including Living Alone) for the Population 65 Years and Over," Summary File 2 (2000), PCT 21.

U.S. Department of Health and Human Services. *Health, United States, 1999: Health and Aging Chartbook* (1999). DDHS Publication number (PHS)99-1232-1.

Viorst, Judith. *Necessary Losses* (New York: Simon and Schuster, 1986).

Willard, Ann. "Cultural Scripts for Mothering." In *Mapping the Moral Domain: A Contribution of Women's Thinking to Psychological Theory and Education,* ed. Carol Gilligan (Cambridge, MA: Harvard University Press, 1988), pp. 225–43.

Winnicott, D. W. *The Family and Individual Development* (London: Tavistock Publications, 1965).

INDEX

abandonment, feelings of, 124–30
abusive parents, 47–48, 177–79
access, sibling, 150
activities of daily living, need for help
    with, 6
Adelman, Ron, 168–69
adolescence, separation process during, 17
affection, lack of, in childhood, 7–8, 66
African-Americans, 167–69, 174–82, 227
aggression, 60
    turned inward, 87
Alcoholics Anonymous, 12, 34, 239
alcoholism, 222–24
    parental, 34–38, 75, 76, 79, 80, 206, 221,
        234–42, 251
Alzheimer's disease, 96–97, 101, 106, 171,
        183–87
    anger at parent with, 15, 98, 110
    memory-enhancing medication for, 91,
        92
    nursing home care for, 97–98, 229
    siblings and, 146, 224–25
ambivalence, 5, 23–24, 41–42, 208
    of daughters toward mothers, 189, 199,
        200
    guilt over, 86
    of parents toward their parents, 62
    tolerating, 247–48
anger, 5, 9, 55–83, 189, 212, 246
    accepting legitimacy of, 22

at controlling behavior, 50
childhood feelings of, 7
forgiving yourself for, 15–16
getting over, by setting limits, 75–82
guilt and, 56–57, 95–105, 232, 248–49
hanging on to, 69–75
identifying triggers of, 59–60
and inability to set limits, 31, 53
at mentally ill parent, 130–31, 133–34,
        136, 137
sibling rivalry and, 40
stress of, physical manifestations of, 14
uncovering sources of, 62–68
working through, 60–61, 68–69, 82, 242
anxiety, 27, 28, 85
    dementia and, 133
    guilt and, 109
    insecure attachment and, 29
Aricept, 91, 92
arthritis, 86, 121
Asian-Americans, 167–68
assisted living facilities, 41, 44, 58, 76, 89,
        90, 132, 136, 171, 195–96
    parent's refusal to move into, 130–32
attachment, 185
    balancing separation and, 18, 19
    insecure, 29, 31, 37–38, 171, 182

baby boomers, care of elderly parents
        by, 9

"bad daughter," image of self as, 20–21
"Bad Mommy Taboo," 5
Bank, Stephen P., 141, 150, 155
Beattie, Melody, 39
bed-wetting, 8
bipolar disorder, 18, 19, 130, 131, 134–35, 234, 242
blackmail, emotional, 118
boundaries, 17
   secure, 31
   see also limits, setting
Bowlby, John, 255n1
Brooklyn College, 215
Brothers and Sisters: How They Shape Our Lives (Leder), 141

California, University of, 212
cancer, 50, 65, 76, 80, 86, 130, 131, 147–49, 190, 206, 207, 240
Caribbean-Americans, 166, 167
cataract surgery, 65, 122–23
Catholics, 50, 79, 235
Chapin, Harry, 233
childhood
   abandonment during, 125–26
   death of parent during, 147–51, 159
   identifying hurts from, 59–60
   insecure attachment during, 29
   limit setting during, 30–31
   with mentally ill parent, 134–35
   of parents, painful experiences during, 47–48, 60–61, 66–67, 102, 204–205, 214
   reemergence of feelings from, 6–9, 21–22, 65–66, 71–72, 92–93, 201, 245
   separation process during, 17–19
   sibling relationships in, 141, 149–51
   working out unresolved issues from, 10, 15
Chinese families, 166
codependency, 38–39
Codependent No More (Beattie), 39
congestive heart failure, 32, 210, 215
controlling behavior, 50, 63
   cultural scripts and, 173, 184
   limit setting by spouse on, 123–24

Cornell University, Weill Medical College of, 168
cultural scripts, 165–88
   of African-Americans, 167–69, 174–82
   of Italian-Americans, 167, 170–74, 187
   of Latinos, 166–70, 182–88

Dance of Anger, The (Lerner), 56
daughters, 13–14, 189–217
   cultural scripts of, 166–70, 183
   "good," 11, 32, 87
   limit setting by, 143
   reawakening of childhood feelings of, 245
   reciprocity of parents and, 49–53
   relationships of fathers and, 208–17
   relationships of mothers and, 189–207, 215–16
   separation issues of, 18–22
   spouses' response to caregiving by, 124
   sibling relationships of, see siblings
deinstitutionalization, 6
dementia, 24, 69, 76, 132, 167, 168, 182, 201–202
   see also Alzheimer's disease
dependency, childhood feelings of, 70, 71, 83
depression, 80, 128, 204
   in childhood, 149
   cultural scripts and, 171, 173, 188
   guilt and, 91, 173
   of parents, 18–19, 63, 90, 101–102, 193, 205
   of siblings, 78, 103–104
   see also bipolar disorder
deprivation, sense of, 34, 36, 103
DeSalo, Louise, 202–203, 208
developmental stage, caregiving as, 9–10, 15, 24
diabetes, 176
Diaz, Michael, 169, 170
displacement, 22–23
distancing from parents, 28–29
dreams, 19
   recurrent, 104
drug addiction, parental, 39, 42,48

Eisenhower, Dwight D., 211–12
emotional blackmail, 118
empathy, lack of, 46, 130
enabling behavior, 34, 25
    of spouses, 118–20
envy, parental, 85–86, 103
Erikson, Erik, 253*n*6
ethnicity, 10, 165–70
    see also specific ethnic groups
expectations, 57
    gender, *see* gender expectations
    guilt about failing to meet, 85

family script, 147
family structure, changes in, 116
feeding tubes, decisions about, 99–100,
        103, 104, 109
feeling rules, 5, 7
fertility, decline in, 6
forgiveness, 214–15
    of alcoholic father, 234–42
    of neediness, 67–68
    of yourself, 109–11, 138, 231
Freud, Sigmund, 60, 87, 204

gender expectations, 10, 220
    changes in, 115–16
    in cultural scripts, 166
    in employment versus caregiving,
        13–14
    parental favoritism and, 10, 11
    role reversals in, 132
    in sibling relationships, 141–46, 159
geographic proximity, 144
good-enough parents, 17, 58
"good mother," 5
    aunt as, 69, 70
    "bad child" self-image and, 20–21, 82
Grant, Linda, 189, 200–202
Greenberg, Vivian, 142–43, 246
guilt, 5, 50, 56, 84–111, 138, 246–47
    anger and, 56–57, 95–105, 110, 232,
        248–49
    childhood feelings of, 7
    depression and, 91, 173
    about envious parents, 85–86, 103
    and forgiving yourself, 109–11

"shoulds" and, 85, 87, 88–95, 110
    of special child, 86–87, 105–11
    separation, 85, 87, 94, 110
    spouses and alleviation of, 117
    stress of, physical manifestations of, 14

Hasidic Jews, 2
heart disease, 130
    see also congestive heart failure
Heritage Day Health Centers (Columbus,
        Ohio), 12
hip, broken, 32
Hispanics, *see* Latinos

Indians, East, 166
introjects, 199
Irish-Americans, 166
isolation, emotional, 150–51
Italian-Americans, 49, 57, 87, 124, 167,
        170–74, 187

Jews, 8–9, 167, 169, 211
    Hasidic, 2

Kahn, Michael D., 141, 150, 155
Klein, Melanie, 255*n*17
knee-replacement surgery, 130, 133,
        136

Latinos, 2, 166–70, 182–88
Leder, Jane Mersky, 141
Lerner, Harriet, 56
life accounting, 251–52
life expectancy, increase in, 6, 9
limits, setting, 16, 27–54, 154, 248, 251
    cultural scripts and, 174
    getting over anger by, 75–82
    insecure attachment and, 29, 31
    reciprocity and, 49–53
    resistance to, 151–52, 159
    with self-centered parent, 41–49
    separation and, 17–24, 33–34
    spouses and, 118–24, 136–39
loss, feelings of, 10, 55–56
    during old age, 58
lupus, 125, 184
Lustbader, Wendy, 47

macular degeneration, 171
Mahler, Margaret, 254*n*14
Maimonides Hospital (Brooklyn), 2
manic-depressive disorder, *see* bipolar
        disorder
Medicare, 32
memory loss, 28, 30, 56
    see also Alzheimer's disease; dementia
mental illness
    of parents, 18, 19, 39, 130–32, 134–39,
        178, 222, 234–35, 238–39, 242,
        251
    of siblings, 78, 103–104
Mills, C. Wright, 244
mirroring, 40
Moody, Rick, 218–20
moral guilt, 86
Moran, Michael, 27
Mount Sinai Medical Center, 169
Mourning and Melancholia (Freud), 204

National Family Caregivers Association
        (NFCA), 13, 14
Necessary Losses (Viorst), 38
neediness
    coming to grips with, 51, 248
    drowning in, 27–28, 30, 35, 49, 72–73,
        206
    forgiving, 67–68
    insecure vs. secure attachment and,
        31–32
    warding off, 205–207
neurotic guilt, 87, 110
New York Academy of Medicine, 168
New York Department of the Aging, 88
nursing homes, 6, 76, 84, 117, 158–59,
        226, 229
    Alzheimer's patients in, 97–98, 104, 229
    cultural differences in attitudes toward,
        166–67, 174–75, 181, 182, 185,
        187
    spending time with parents in,
        229–32

oedipal issues, 216
One True Thing (Quindlen), 12–13,
        202

only children, spouses of, 130–39
osteoporosis, 41

panic attacks, 38
paranoia, 42
phobias, 29, 153–54
post-traumatic stress syndrome, 236–37
postpartum depression, 103–104
powerlessness, feelings of, 71–72
psychoanalytic theory, 19, 40, 87, 199
Puerto Ricans, 169, 182–88
Purple America (Moody), 218–20

Quindlen, Anna, 12–13, 202

rage, 34, 36
reciprocity, 40–53, 122
recovery movement, 38–39
regression, 21–22, 74, 138, 188
regret, feelings of, 43
religious beliefs, 52–53
    cultural scripts and, 179–80
Remind Me Who I Am Again (Grant),
        200–202
remorse, feelings of, 10
resentment, 47
    guilt and, 103
    parental, 102
    toward siblings, 145
resistance, 22–24
*Respecting Your Limits While Caring for Elderly
        Parents* (Greenberg), 142
respite care, 226
Roman Catholic Church, 22
Rubin, Lillian, 199–202

sacrifices, making, 36
sadness, feelings of, 10, 43
school phobias, 29
Secunda, Victoria, 5, 22
self, sense of
    consolidation of, 10
    loss of, Alzheimer's disease and, 184
    mirroring and, 40
    moral guilt and, 86
    separation and, 17
senile dementia, *see* dementia

separation, 9, 15, 17–24, 33–34, 222–24
  acceptance of, 252
  ambivalence and, 200
  codependency and, 39
  failed, of parents from their parents, 61–62
  guilt about, 85, 87, 94, 110
  from image of self as "bad daughter," 20–21
  and reemergence of childhood feelings, 21–22
  resistance to, 22–24, 71–74, 153, 171–72
  working out issues of, 51–52
sexual abuse, 178–79
Sheehy, Gail, 13
Shepard, Sam, 21
"shoulds," 85, 87, 88–95, 110
Sibling Bond, The (Bank and Kahn), 141, 150, 155
siblings, 6, 10–11, 42, 45, 81, 140–61
  acceptance of, 232–33
  acting out by, 33, 37
  alliance against abusive mother of, 211, 212, 214
  conflicted feelings toward, 89–90
  creating connections among, through caregiving, 147–60
  cultural scripts and, 172–73, 175–77, 184–85
  death of, 126–27
  failure as caregivers of, 224–25
  in family script, 147
  gendered division of labor between, 141–46, 159
  limit setting by, 28
  mentally ill, 78, 103–104
  mutuality among, 160–61
  parents', 62–63, 77
  problems of, 78
  relationships with, 15
  resentment toward, 78–79
  rivalry with, 33, 35–37, 40, 141
  sharing of care by, 63–65, 68, 190–91, 194, 215
  of special child, 105–108
  suicide of, 203–204
  support for primary caregivers from, 122, 123

Silent Passage, The (Sheehy), 13
social class, 10
sons, 13–14, 218–43
  cultural scripts of, 166, 168–74
  limit setting by, 143
  relationships of mothers and, 218–28, 242–43
  relationships of fathers and, 223–24, 228–43
  separation issues of, 19–20
  spouses' response to caregiving by, 124
  sibling relationships of, see siblings
specialness, feelings of
  cultural scripts and, 185–86, 188
  and disowning of siblings, 165
  guilt and, 86–87, 105–11
  and relationship with father, 209–10
  wish for, 153, 216
Spock, Benjamin, 233
spouses, 115–39
  abandonment by, 124–30
  and changing gender expectations, 115–16
  division of labor between, 142
  ill, caretaking needs of, 152–54, 158, 183
  and limit setting, 118–24, 136–39
  of only children, importance of, 130–39
  participation in caregiving by, 225–27
Stevenson, Adlai, 211
strokes, 105, 229
  memory loss from, 28
suicide, 203–204, 223, 224
  attempted, 78, 135, 238, 239
surgery
  deterioration after, 95–96
  pneumonia following, 75–76
  recovery from, 63–65

Tangled Lives (Rubin), 199
toilet training, 30–31
True West (Shepard), 21
trust, rebuilding, 129–30

valve replacement surgery, 63–64
ventilator, removal of, 99, 105

Vertigo (DeSalvo), 202–203
Vietnam War, 212, 233
violence, parental, 41–44
Viorst, Judith, 38
Visiting Nurses Association, 158

Walson, Bonnie, 12
When You and Your Mother Can't Be Friends
    (Secunda), 22
Winnicott, D. W., 254*n*15
World War II, 78, 236–37

ABOUT THE AUTHOR

Roberta Satow is chairperson of the Department of Sociology at Brooklyn College, a senior member of the National Psychological Association for Psychoanalysis, and a practicing psychoanalyst in New York City. She has taught the sociology of gender at Brooklyn College and Columbia Teachers College for the last twenty years. In addition to her book *Gender and Social Life*, she has written many articles on sociological and psychoanalytic subjects that have appeared in numerous journals and magazines including *Psychoanalytic Review*, *Partisan Review* and *Psychology Today*.